The Herbal Healing Bible

Discover traditional herbal remedies to treat everyday ailments and common conditions the natural way

Jade Britton

CHARTWELL BOOKS, INC.

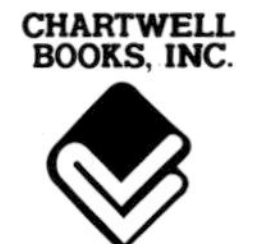

A QUANTUM BOOK

This edition published in 2012 by
CHARTWELL BOOKS, INC.
A division of BOOK SALES INC.,
276 Fifth Avenue, Suite 206
New York, New York 10001
USA

ISBN 13: 978-0-7858-2965-2

Produced by
Quantum Publishing Ltd
The Old Brewery
6 Blundell Street
London N7 9BH

QUMTHHB

Assistant Editor: Jo Morley
Managing Editor: Samantha Warrington
Production Manager: Rohana Yusof
Publisher: Sarah Bloxham

Packaged by Gulmohur

Printed in China by Midas Printing International Ltd.

Quantum would like to thank and acknowledge the following for supplying the pictures reproduced in this book:

Shutterstock: p22, 24, 25, 60, 62, 77, 79, 83, 92, 102, 104, 113, 115, 116, 117, 122, 125, 136, 140, 150, 158, 162,

iStock: p50, 54, 68, 74, 75, 95, 99, 101, 106, 118, 120, 124, 126, 133, 144, 154,

Corbis: p13, 107, 108, 110, 135

Getty: p9

Pat Brindley: p168, 173, 176, 180, 189, 191, 194, 196, 198

Horticultural Photographic Collection: p166, 167, 169, 170, 172, 174, 175, 177, 179, 182, 186, 188, 192, 193, 197, 199, 200, 202, 204, 205, 206, 207, 208, 209, 210, 211, 212, 213, 214, 215

The Image Bank: p35, 56, 81, 82, 89, 97, 109

Peter McHoy: p171, 178, 183, 184, 185, 203

Photos Horticultural Picture Library: p190

Photo/Nats Inc. p187, 195, 201

Pictor International: p26, 53, 61, 96, 128, 142 143, 156, 161

Tony Stone Images: p10, 15, 28 58, 65, 69, 76, 87,119, 139, 146, 148

While every effort has been made to credit contributors, Quantum would like to apologize should there have been any omissions or errors.

The material in this book originally appeared in *The Complete Book of Herbal Remedies.*

Contents

Foreword

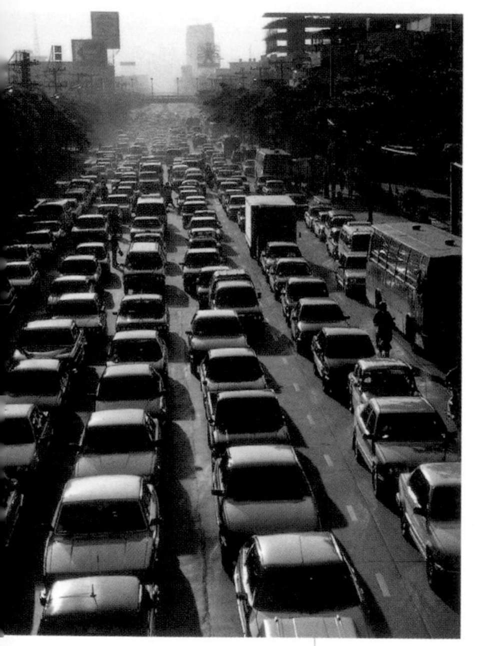

Above Pollution caused by our consumer-driven society is threatening our health and the health of the planet as a whole.

We are living in a time of great diversity, change, and confusion. We are overwhelmed by choices of healing systems, concepts, and treatment techniques. Some people feel that herbal medicine is just one of a variety of alternative therapies. It is far from that, since it is used by up to 80 per cent of the world's population for their health care needs. Herbal medicine does not oppose conventional medicine, but it can be used as a first-line therapy in a more natural healing fashion. In fact, many of today's modern or "miracle" drugs have grown from the roots of herbalism. But even though modern medicine has its basis in herbalism, often a drug is over-refined and may have lost some of the other components that complement or prevent side-effects.

Plant medicine has been used in a therapeutic fashion since antiquity in the healing of the body, mind, and spirit. This philosophy is our heritage. Herbal medicine uses a holistic approach to healing and shows ways of enhancement, rather than just treating symptoms. Symptoms are our body's way of signalling that something is wrong and needs attention. By selecting natural methods, we choose to become more aware, connected, and conscious.

This is a time of limited financial medical resources, and restricted availability of medical care. Herbal medicine is in the perfect position to fill the gap and treat both simple and more complicated medical problems. Although the theory of herbal medicine is grounded in historical facts, it is far from folklore and there is clinical and scientific research to document its efficacy. This book outlines the many ways to use botanicals in healing in a practical and useful format. Herbs can be used as a tonic, as treatment, and as a preventative. The advantages of using an inexpensive, effective, and less toxic substance are clearly beneficial.

"What is health and healing all about?", is fast becoming one major question for the 21st century. Protection of the rain forest and fighting pollution is vital if we are to prevent important healing plants from becoming extinct. Herbal medicine is thought to act by creating a homeostatic (metabolically balanced) healing process, rather than a suppressive one. By doing so, it promotes a balance toward health. Herbal medicine is therefore not anti-technology, but rather for self-care. We must integrate herbal therapies with conventional and complementary treatment. This holistic care gives us the knowledge and awareness to use appropriate botanical medicines. It also gives us the understanding of the relationship between ourselves, our environment, and each other. Then as we heal ourselves, we can heal the planet.

Edward J. Linkner M.D.

Below By protecting the natural world we live in, and taking care not to deplete the bounty it shares with us, we can begin to improve our own health and well-being.

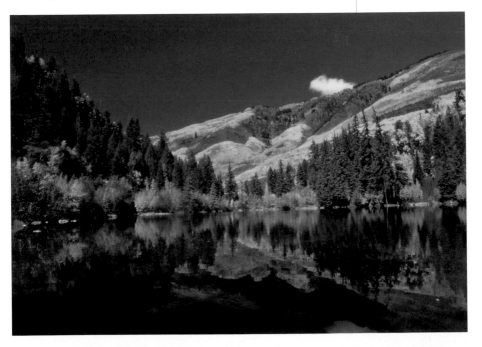

Introduction

The magic of plants has touched most of us. We marvel at their simple beginnings as a seed, the pattern of their unfolding leaves, and the fragrance and delicacy of their flowers. A field of wild flowers and grasses or a forest of leafy trees can uplift us.

What is Herbalism?

Herbalism is the use of plants as medicines for healing. Its traditions are as old as mankind itself, and until the 18th century it was used as the most common form of medical treatment in Europe and North America. Today, in tribal cultures and among countries with Eastern traditions, such as China and India, medicinal herbs are still widely used. In more conventional medicine, pharmaceutical companies and doctors rely on plants as the basis of many drugs.

Early Herbalism

The first written herbal records date back well over 5,000 years, to the Sumerians, who described the use and actions of plants such as laurel, caraway, and thyme. The ancient Egyptians used garlic, coriander, mint, castor oil, and opium. References in the Old Testament also speak of the use of herbal medicines.

Ancient Chinese Herbals

Chinese herbal medicine dates back to the 3rd century BC, with manuscripts found in *Ma Wang Dui* Tomb Three in Hunan province. These contained references to more than 250 medicinal substances and how to use them in prescriptions. The *Yellow Emperor's Inner Classic*, compiled over 2,000 years ago, discusses the philosophical questions of health, illness, and the relationship of the human body to the cosmos. It also contains suggestions for herbs, acupuncture, diet, and exercise which are still relevant today.

The traditional Chinese herbal has increased since then with the integration of substances from China's folk medicine and from other parts of Southeast Asia, India, and the Middle East.

Greek and Roman Concepts

Ancient Greek and Roman medical practices are the basis for conventional medicine used in Western society today. Hippocrates, the Greek physician and "father of medicine," advocated the use of a few simple herbal drugs, along with fresh air, rest, and a healthy diet to aid the body in strengthening its own "life force" to eliminate its problems. Galen, an influentical Roman physician, believed in using larger doses of the remedies, including plant, animal, and mineral substances, as the means to heal diseases. The first European treatise on the properties and uses of medicinal herbs was *De Materia Medica*, written in the 1st century AD by the Greek physician Dioscorides. It was used well into the 17th century.

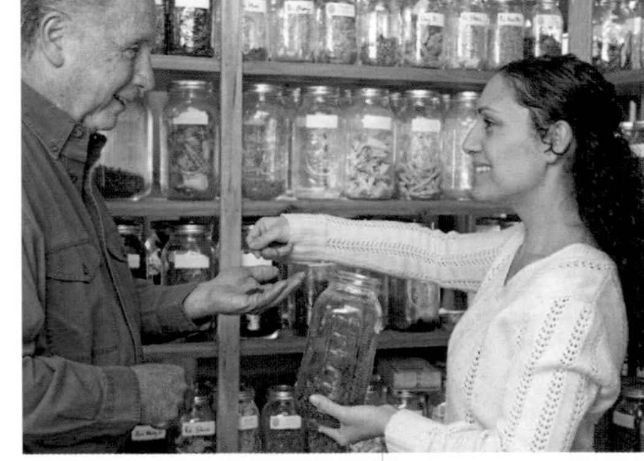

Above The use of plants as medicines predates written human history. In 2001, researchers identified 122 compounds used in modern medicine which were derived from "ethnomedical" plant sources.

The Middle Ages

The use of plants for medicines was common practice during the Middle Ages. The early Christian church discouraged this, preferring faith healing. However, the diligent work of the monks preserved many Greek medical manuscripts, and the monasteries, with their herb gardens, became local centers for herbal treatment. Folk medicine continued the use of herbal traditions, with knowledge held by midwives and "wise women." Fear and superstition were rife, with many magical properties attached to herbal medicine. Ultimately this led to the persecution and death of many women, healers, and so-called witches. The use of herbs was passed on through apprenticeship and word of mouth. Consequently, a great loss of herbal tradition occurred during the Inquisition, when many herbalists were put to death.

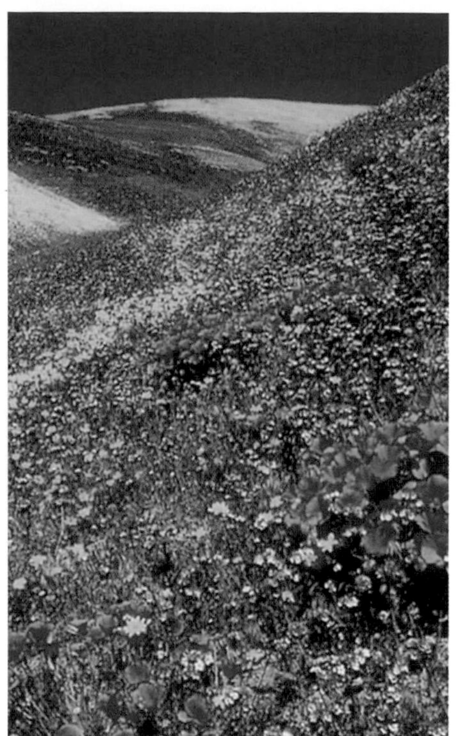

Above Many of the plants used in herbal treatments grow in the wild around the world.

Western Herbalism

Despite the move in the 19th century toward the use of sophisticated drugs, 80 per cent of the world's population still depends on medicines derived from traditional plant remedies. The recognition of the importance of ancient herbal traditions is increasing as people seek to find a greater understanding of themselves and their connection with the world around them.

The Balancing Nature of Herbs

Plants take up substances from the earth and convert them into vitamins, minerals, carbohydrates, proteins, and fats that our bodies use for nourishment and healing. By using the whole plant or herb, we take in all the vital ingredients it carries. Most herbs contain several active substances, one of which usually dominates and determines its choice as a remedy. However the other healing aspects of the herb should not be overlooked because they will help the body to assimilate its benefits and buffer any potential side-effects.

Herb Combinations

Herbs work synergistically, so combining them enhances each herb's properties, helping to bring greater healing to the body. For example, a good mixture to help induce sleep combines passiflora, valerian, and hops. All three herbs have relaxant properties, but passiflora specializes in aiding sleep, valerian relaxes muscle tension, and hops have a marked effect on relaxing the nervous system.

Chinese Herbalism

Chinese herbs are rarely used on their own; more commonly they are used in combination to form a Chinese prescription. The use of many herbs helps to achieve a balance within the prescription, and ensures that it enters the part of the body that needs healing. Herbs are described in terms of temperature, taste, what they do in the body, and whether they affect the *yin, yang, qi,* or blood.

Yin and *Yang*

The concept of *yin* and *yang* is part of traditional Chinese philosophy. It states that all systems of the universe consist of two conflicting yet interdependent energies from which all forms of creation came. The nature of *yang* is hot, bright, upward, and active, embodying the more masculine energy. The *yin* holds the cool, moist, inward, and nourishing qualities, which are the more feminine principles. For example, astragalus is a *yang* herb used to warm, strengthen and raise the *qi,* or energy. Lycium fruit is a *yin* herb whose actions go deep into the body, working to restore depleted functions as well as to prevent further deterioration.

Qi and Blood

In terms of Chinese medicine, *qi* is an energy which manifests simultaneously on the physical, emotional, and spiritual levels, and is in a constant state of change. It is the vital force of life. Blood is seen as a denser, more material, form of *qi. Qi* generates, moves, and holds blood, yet blood nourishes *qi,* or, as the Chinese saying goes, "Blood is the mother of *qi.*" Ginseng (*ren shen*) tonifies the *qi* of the body, including that of the lungs, digestion, and heart. The herb Chinese angelica (*dang gui*) tonifies and moves the blood (it actually strengthens the *qi* of the blood).

Combining Western and Chinese Herbalism

In this book, remedies include both traditional Chinese and Western herbal suggestions. They can be used together safely as long as you consider any cautions and contraindications, and use the safe dosages (see pp.26–27). Many traditional Chinese remedies are given as patent remedies, and in their pill form can be used easily and safely over a period of time. Western herbal teas can be drunk at the same time to help treat any ailment. Herbal tinctures are another easy way that you can combine Chinese and Western herbs.

Thinking Holistically

By recognizing that there is a link between our mind and body, and to the world around us, we start to understand the importance of holistic health. By healing ourselves through working closely with gifts from nature, we learn to care for the environment.

Herbs and the Environment

Our ecological awareness is much needed to avert a crisis on the planet on which we depend for life. Increasing pollution, the destruction of the rain forests, and climate change could all have a potentially disastrous effect on us. Some herbs, which are more commonly seen as weeds, are remarkably resilient. Any gardener knows that nettles, dock, and couchgrass proliferate in most conditions. However, the more obscure healing plants are being lost as their environment is destroyed. Nature's gifts for healing are disappearing as we wipe out traditional tribal societies, losing their knowledge, lands, and the plants they grow.

Living in Harmony with Nature

We need to find a way of living in harmony with the world around us to ensure a good quality of life. Plants provide us with oxygen through photosynthesis, as well as food and drink, shelter, wood for coal and fuel, and medicines. From us they receive carbon dioxide, help with pollination, and bacteria to break down dead remains and return their substances into the soil, which is the birthplace of new life. As we strengthen our life force through connection with the plants and the world around us, we become more aware of our own vitality (or lack of it) and can find healing for ourselves.

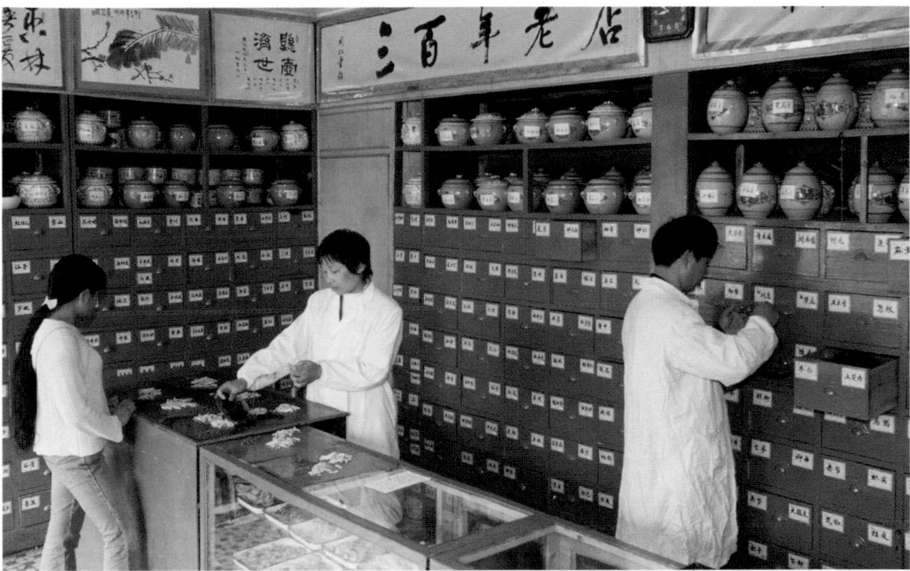

Above Staff at work in a traditional Chinese herbalist.

The "Life Force"

The concept of the "life force" is central to the philosophy of holistic healing. It is the essence that helps the body to heal itself. It is known in Chinese medicine as *qi*, and in other systems of medicine as the vital energy, or *prana*. In a holistic approach, illness occurs when there is a disturbance within this life force. Symptoms of an illness help us to identify what we need in our lives to recover and restore our own healing energy.

The Body in Health

Childhood, or a long holiday, may have included moments when we felt a strong spark of life. Everyday life puts its demands on us, and we cope with them, putting aside the minor complaints of our bodies. It is when these complaints stop us from doing what we want to do that we seek help. By living in an unpolluted environment, eating a healthy diet, taking physical exercise, finding peace of mind and a positive attitude, you can do a great deal to restore good health. Herbal medicine offers much, helping us to take responsibility for our own health, and offering simple treatments. Today, in North America, increasing numbers of holistic physicians combine conventional and alternative therapies in the prevention and treatment of diseases.

Environmental Factors

A pollution-free environment is hard to find these days, and is not practical for everyone. It is important to know the effect of pollution on your body. Some people are obviously more sensitive, such as asthmatics, and they need to take extra care when pollution levels are high. Herbal treatments may help to boost immunity and calm reactions to environmental factors, but a long-term environmental solution is also needed.

Diet

Food is an essential part of life, and a good diet goes a long way in preventing serious illness. A wholefood diet of preferably organic foods will help support good health. Fresh fruit and vegetables are necessary to supply essential vitamins and minerals and the roughage needed to clear wastes from the body. Avoid eating excessive amounts of foods high in refined sugars and flours, such as cakes, cookies, and candy, as well as drinking coffee, tea, alcohol, and smoking.

Exercise

Our society has become more technological; the physical exercise that was once part of everyday life has been replaced by modern conveniences and exercise has become an optional form of recreation. This is fine, but we must make a point of exercising because it helps us to relax and release tension, build up muscle tone, and strengthen both our heart and lungs. It encourages the circulation of the blood and lymph systems, so all parts of the body are warm, and our immunity is enhanced.

Peace of Mind

Our physical, emotional, and mental health are strongly connected. Many physical ailments, such as headaches, digestive complaints, and low immunity, are linked with stress. There are many herbal teas, baths, and oils listed throughout this book that help us to relax and let go of tensions. It may also be important to talk through difficult

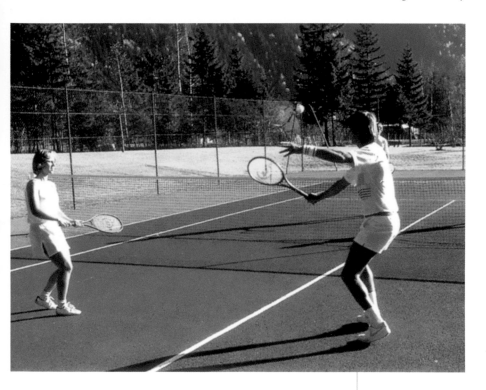

Above Exercise strengthens the cardiovascular system and provides a good release for everyday stress and tension.

situations, and counseling can help with this. Relaxation through yoga, meditation, and *t'ai chi* can be beneficial for restoring peace of mind; as can simple pleasures like gardening, singing, and walking.

Spirituality

Spirituality is the belief in the greater good that is within all of us. Although in these times it can be difficult to carry this belief, the other option leaves us open to negativity, pessimism, and cynicism. A positive state of mind, which carries with it hope, an openness to different ways of being, and compassion for others and ourselves, helps to encourage good feelings about life.

Deciding on an Herbal Treatment

There are many different ways of using herbs to provide a wide variety of treatments. Herbs can be taken as teas, wines, and syrups,

Healing the body as a whole

Symptoms caused by emotional difficulties may not respond to herbal treatments. Resolving your problems with a therapist or counselor should enable you to respond more freely to the treatments.

A positive mental attitude, an openness to different ways of being, and compassion for others and ourselves, help to encourage good feelings about life.

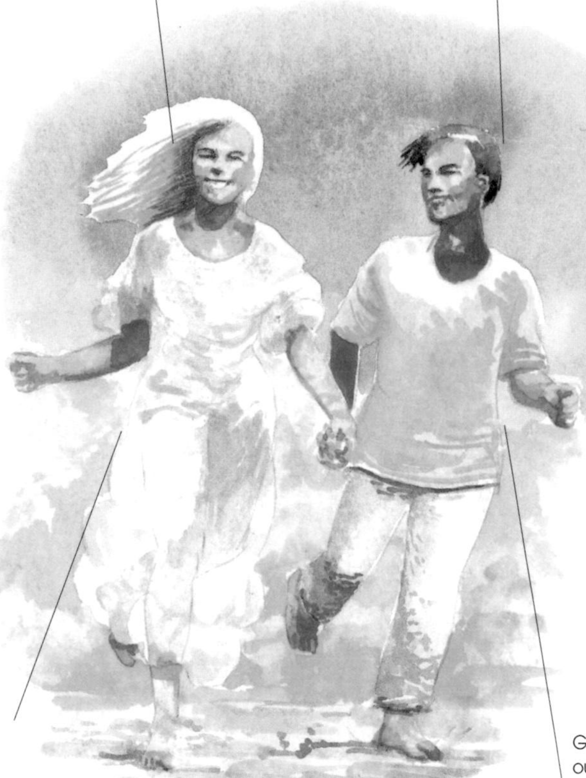

Adopting a healthier lifestyle and learning to relax are an essential part of holistic treatment.

Good health lies in our own hands. Herbal remedies can help us to treat minor ailments before they develop into more serious problems.

or used externally as baths, creams, and lotions. The simplest and most common method is an herbal tea. Because of their increasing popularity, several of the more widely known herbal teas, such as peppermint, camomile, and rosehip, can be bought in supermarkets. If you do not enjoy their taste, try the peppermint or camomile as an essential oil in your bath!

Herbs for Prevention

Taking herbs to prevent illness and ailments is both effective and useful. Garlic and echinacea help to boost the immune system, and are especially helpful if there is a tendency to colds or infections during the winter. If you are prone to anxiety, and are aware that you are facing a particularly difficult time, try drinking camomile tea to help you relax. Use lavender oil in a bath or on your pillow to help you sleep at night so that you get a good night's rest and can cope better. Herbs can be used at the first sign of a complaint to avoid a more serious illness. Drink a hot peppermint tea with honey and a few slices of ginger root with the first sniffle of a cold, or a hot tea of boneset to ward off flu symptoms.

Using Herbs Safely

Herbal medicine, like any other medicine, deserves care and respect. The Herbal Directory (see pp.164–215) lists the herbs most frequently used in this book, along with any cautions or contraindications. Take the time to look at these when you have decided on the herbs best suited for your treatment. The dosages are also given for each herb, and must be closely followed. Standard dosages for infusions, decoctions, tinctures, wines, baths, inhalations, and Chinese patent remedies are given in the Herbal Methods chapter (see pp.20–47). Remember that dosages will vary with age, so children and the elderly should take less than adults (see pp.26–27). If a woman is breastfeeding, any herb she is taking will be passed on to the baby in her milk. It is therefore important to seek professional advice. If you are taking homeopathic remedies, you should consult a homeopath or herbal practitioner before beginning any herbal treatment. If you are in any doubt about using an herb, consult a professional herbalist.

How to use this Book

This book is divided into three main sections. You may choose to read parts of it for general interest, or consult it for treatment for different ailments. It is a reference for herbs that may be used simply and effectively to treat a wide variety of complaints. It seeks to give you a greater understanding of how the body works, and how to use herbal medicine.

THE BODY AND HOW TO TREAT IT

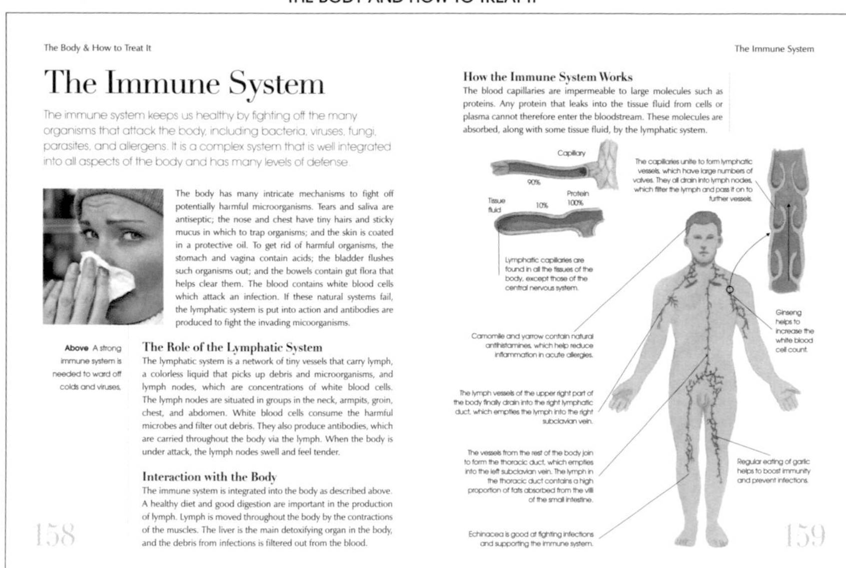

The Body & How to Treat It

The Immune System

The immune system keeps us healthy by fighting off the many organisms that attack the body, including bacteria, viruses, fungi, parasites, and allergens. It is a complex system that is well integrated into all aspects of the body and has many levels of defense.

The body has many intricate mechanisms to fight off potentially harmful microorganisms. Tears and saliva are antiseptic; the nose and chest have tiny hairs and sticky mucus in which to trap organisms; and the skin is coated in a protective oil. To get rid of harmful organisms, the stomach and vagina contain acids; the bladder flushes such organisms out; and the bowels contain gut flora that helps clear them. The blood contains white blood cells which attack an infection. If these natural systems fail, the lymphatic system is put into action and antibodies are produced to fight the invading micoorganisms.

Above A strong immune system is needed to ward off colds and viruses.

The Role of the Lymphatic System

The lymphatic system is a network of tiny vessels that carry lymph, a colorless liquid that picks up debris and microorganisms, and lymph nodes, which are concentrations of white blood cells. The lymph nodes are situated in groups in the neck, armpits, groin, chest, and abdomen. White blood cells consume the harmful microbes and filter out debris. They also produce antibodies, which are carried throughout the body via the lymph. When the body is under attack, the lymph nodes swell and feel tender.

Interaction with the Body

The immune system is integrated into the body as described above. A healthy diet and good digestion are important in the production of lymph. Lymph is moved throughout the body by the contractions of the muscles. The liver is the main detoxifying organ in the body, and the debris from infections is filtered out from the blood.

158

The Immune System

How the Immune System Works

The blood capillaries are impermeable to large molecules such as proteins. Any protein that leaks into the tissue fluid from cells or plasma cannot therefore enter the bloodstream. These molecules are absorbed, along with some tissue fluid, by the lymphatic system.

Capillary
90%
Tissue fluid
10%
Protein 100%
Lymphatic capillaries are found in all the tissues of the body, except those of the central nervous system.
The capillaries unite to form lymphatic vessels, which have large numbers of valves. They all drain into lymph nodes, which filter the lymph and pass it on to further vessels.
Camomile and yarrow contain natural antihistamines, which help reduce inflammation in acute allergies.
Ginseng helps to increase the white blood cell count.
The lymph vessels of the upper right part of the body finally drain into the right lymphatic duct, which empties the lymph into the right subclavian vein.
The vessels from the rest of the body join to form the thoracic duct, which empties into the left subclavian vein. The lymph in the thoracic duct contains a high proportion of fats absorbed from the villi of the small intestine.
Regular eating of garlic helps to boost immunity and prevent infections.
Echinacea is good at fighting infections and supporting the immune system.

159

Herbal Methods

This chapter describes different techniques for preparing herbs, from the making of infusions, or herbal teas, to ointments and creams. It gives useful recipes, such as an iron tonic medicinal wine, and an eyewash for tired eyes. Dosages, which will differ for the various preparations and with the age of the patient, are also given (see pp.26–27), and these must be consulted before using any herbal treatment.

THE HERBAL DIRECTORY

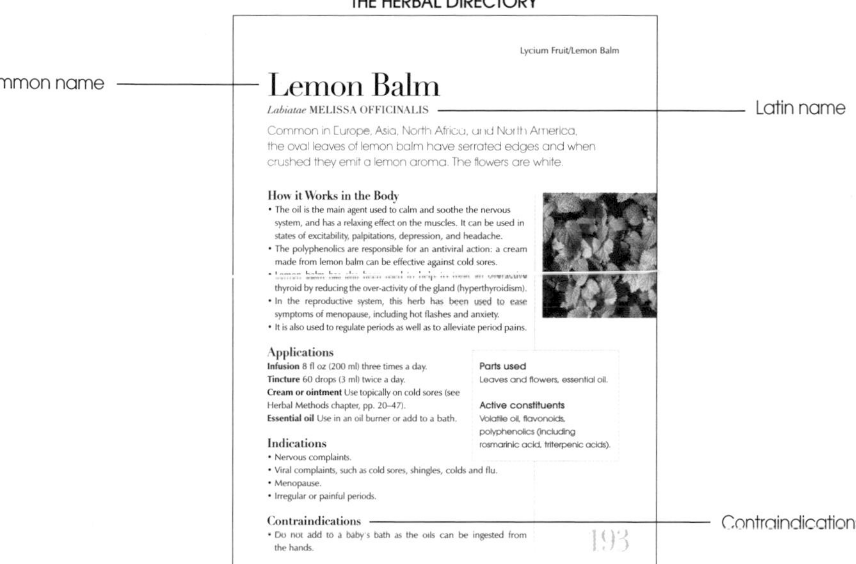

Lycium Fruit/Lemon Balm

Lemon Balm

Labiatae MELISSA OFFICINALIS

Common in Europe, Asia, North Africa, and North America, the oval leaves of lemon balm have serrated edges and when crushed they emit a lemon aroma. The flowers are white.

How it Works in the Body

- The oil is the main agent used to calm and soothe the nervous system, and has a relaxing effect on the muscles. It can be used in states of excitability, palpitations, depression, and headache.
- The polyphenolics are responsible for an antiviral action: a cream made from lemon balm can be effective against cold sores.
- Lemon balm has also been used to help to treat an overactive thyroid by reducing the over-activity of the gland (hyperthyroidism).
- In the reproductive system, this herb has been used to ease symptoms of menopause, including hot flashes and anxiety.
- It is also used to regulate periods as well as to alleviate period pains.

Applications

Infusion 8 fl oz (200 ml) three times a day.
Tincture 60 drops (3 ml) twice a day.
Cream or ointment Use topically on cold sores (see Herbal Methods chapter, pp. 20–47).
Essential oil Use in an oil burner or add to a bath.

Parts used
Leaves and flowers, essential oil.

Active constituents
Volatile oil, flavonoids, polyphenolics (including rosmarinic acid, triterpenic acids).

Indications

- Nervous complaints.
- Viral complaints, such as cold sores, shingles, colds and flu.
- Menopause.
- Irregular or painful periods.

Contraindications

- Do not add to a baby's bath as the oils can be ingested from the hands.

193

The Body and how to Treat it

This chapter divides the body into different systems, looking at how they work and the herbal remedies that can help with their related ailments. Suggestions for preventing illness and keeping the body healthy, as well as advice regarding diet and lifestyle, are also given. Before taking any herbal treatment, check the herbs recommended in the Herbal Directory (pp. 164–215) to ensure correct dosage and that there are no contraindications.

Herbal Directory

This section gives specific information on the herbs recommended in this book, including a brief description of the herb, its use, how to apply it, any contraindications, and appropriate dosages. Herbs used or mentioned in the book but not included in the Directory are described briefly in the Additional Herbs list (pp.216–217). The Glossary (pp.220–221) explains commonly used herbal terminology. This section also includes making remedies from common items found in most kitchens, and suggestions for herbal first-aid treatments.

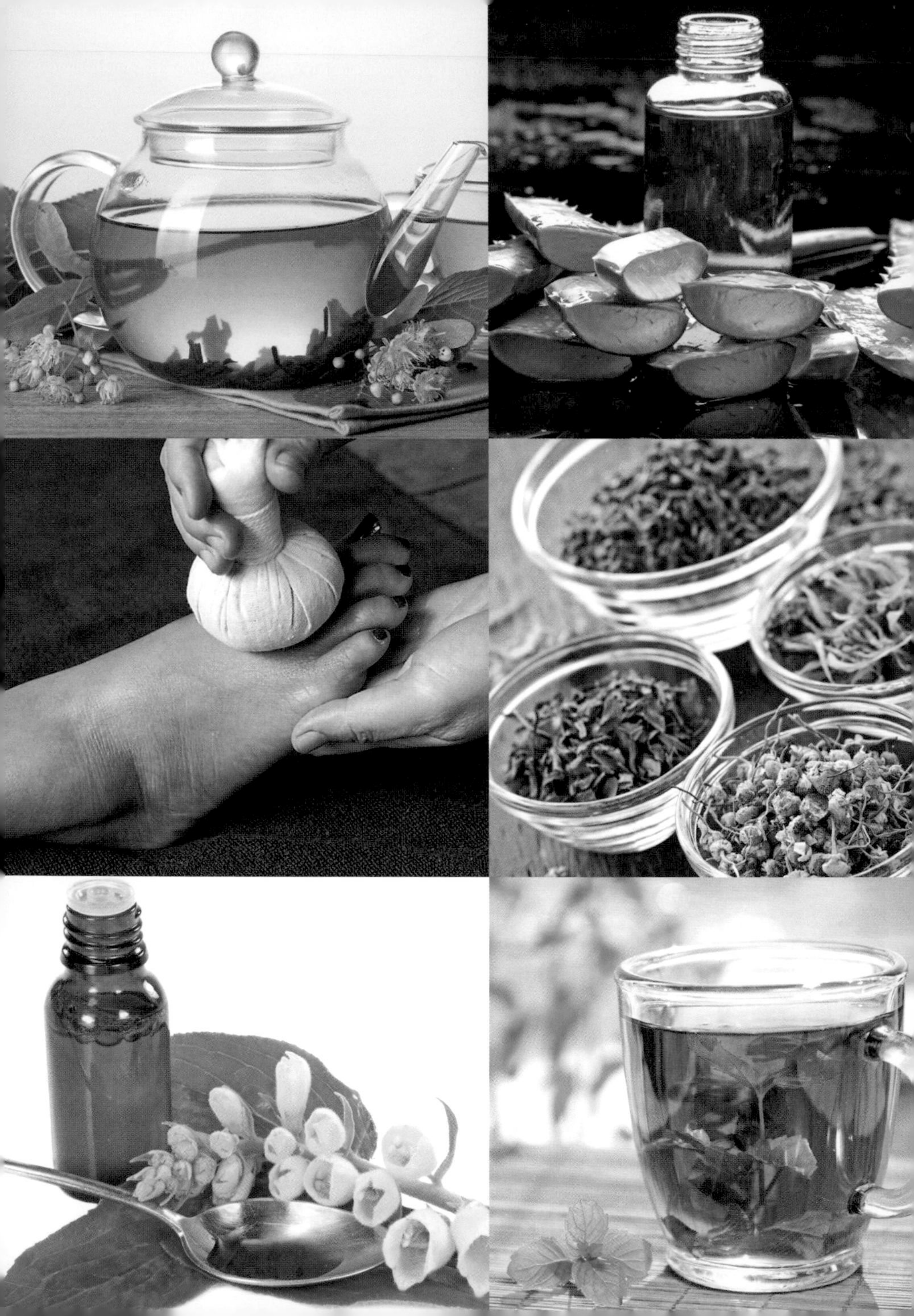

Herbal Methods

This first section deals with the practicalities of using herbal remedies, telling you where to get herbs from, how to select them, grow and pick them and then which parts to use. The chapter then moves on to detailing how to make all the various types of remedy, such as infusions, decoctions and tinctures, and gives information on what the doses should be.

Where to get Herbs

Whether you decide to pick, grow or buy your medicinal herbs, you need to become familiar with all the common dos and don'ts as it's easy to spoil a remedy through being unaware of vital information. Take the time to learn all about herbal preparations and they'll be far more effective.

Choosing Herbs

There are several ways of obtaining herbs. The first is to pick them from the wild, following the guidelines below. This will enable you to have the benefit of gathering fresh herbs, which also can be stored and dried. Second, you can buy dried herbs from a store, or online. Third, you may decide to grow your own herbs. This will give you the advantage of being able to use fresh herbs grown right on your doorstep, enjoying their foliage and scents every day, as well as reaping the medicinal benefits.

Picking Your Own Herbs

There are a few common sense rules about picking your own herbs*:

- It is important to preserve the countryside and never to deplete an area of its natural resources.

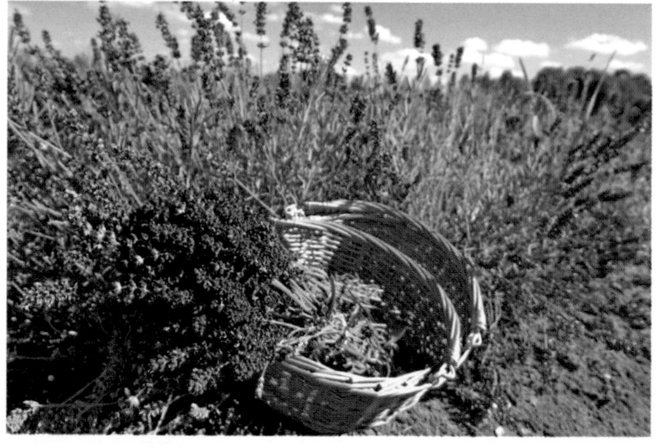

- Do not uproot plants and take them home with you; select just a few specimens for harvesting, and leave the rest to multiply.
- Only harvest common, plentiful plants—the weeds of the countryside—not rare or scarce plants. Check local regulations on gathering herbs.

**Always consult a good field guide to wild plants before attempting to forage in the wild.*

- Always ensure that the plant you are harvesting is the plant you actually require—using a good field guide to wild plants.
- Go on a herb walk with an experienced herbalist, who will identify plants for you and help you learn, too.
- Above all, make sure you are not harvesting a protected species.

Following these rules will ensure that nature's gifts are preserved for everyone to enjoy and benefit from.

Choosing Healthy Herbs

Check that no pesticides or herbicides have been used in the area, and that the plants are not growing close to industrial buildings or busy roads, which may produce waste or pollution. Try to ensure that the herbs are free from animal droppings or insect damage, and are generally healthy, fresh-looking plants.

The Growing Life of the Herb

It is useful to familiarize yourself with the growing life of the plant you are thinking of using. Knowing the plant's habitat and growing season will add greatly to your knowledge of its medicinal value and benefits. Gather the herbs in the morning after the first dew has evaporated, but before the sun is fully on them.

Which Part of the Plant to Use

It is important to find out which part of the plant is best suited for your purpose. For example, while the dandelion leaf acts as a diuretic, and might be useful for those suffering from high blood pressure, the root is suitable for treating the liver, and acts as a mild laxative.

Seasonal Changes

Decide which parts of the plants you intend to use, and check the time of year most suitable for harvesting them. For instance, roots are better harvested in the autumn when the aerial part of the plant has died, leaving the goodness in the roots, to be stored until spring. The leaves of a plant are best harvested in the spring. Flowers, on the other hand, are at their best later in the season. Berries should be picked when they are ripe. Bark should be purchased commercially, as cutting a tree may damage or kill it.

Buying Herbs

You may be able to purchase dried herbs locally or online. Either is likely to be a good source, but be sure to compare the quality by looking at, smelling, and tasting the herbs to ensure value for money. Dried herbs do not have a shelf-life of longer than about a year, so look for color: the flowers should retain some of their color and the leaves should still have some green in them; if calendula looks pale and insipid instead of a glorious orange, it may have been sitting in storage too long. The herbs should also still have a scent. Lastly, test by taste: when infused or decocted you should be able to tell the herbs apart; they should not taste dull or lacking in flavor.

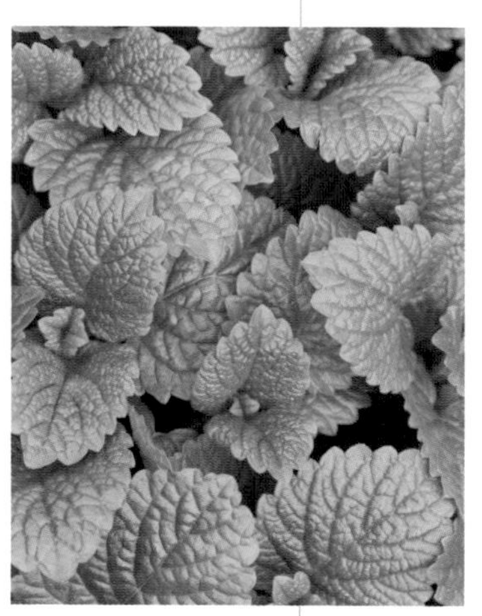

Above The addition of an herbal remedy, such as mint, to a steam inhalation helps to ease congestion, clear mucus, and relieve respiratory stress.

Drying Herbs

You can use herbs fresh, in which case you need to use them quite quickly or they will decay. Alternatively, you can dry the plant carefully in a warm airing cupboard or spread on brown paper on a rack in a warm, shady place. If drying flower heads, such as calendula, or large leaves, set them out so that they do not overlap and air can circulate. Leave them to dry for one to three weeks. If mold appears it means there is too much moisture circulating and you will have to discard the batch and repeat the process. If drying a plant with smaller flowers, such as lavender, or leaves, you can dry them in a paper bag, in bunches of four or five, hung upside down by their stems. Ensure that the bag covers the flower heads or leaves, then secure with an elastic band. Roots should be cleaned and cut into small pieces. Dry them in the oven on a baking tray at about 120°F (50°C) until brittle. If they remain soft, they are retaining moisture, so check them at intervals. Do be patient: too much heat, too fast, may destroy some of the plant's delicate constituents.

Storing Herbs

When the herbs are dry, store them in a clean, dry jar, preferably made of dark glass, and keep them out of the sunlight. When buying dried herbs from a supplier, transfer them into a clean, dry jar with a close-fitting lid. Store in a dry place, away from sunlight.

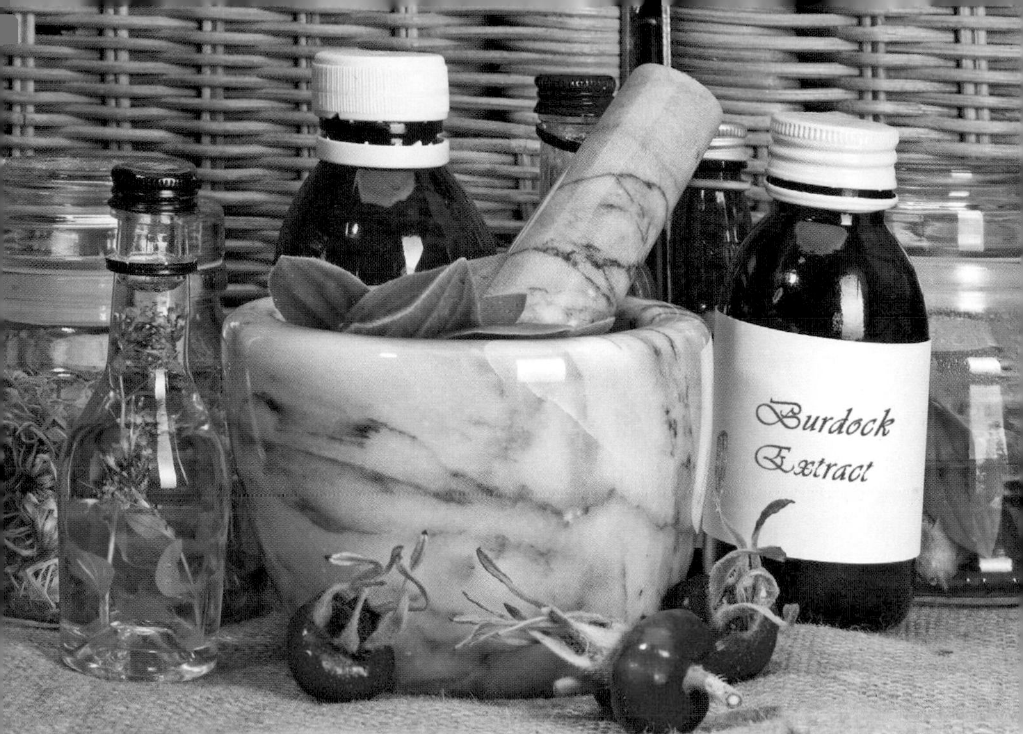

Above You can store and preserve herbs to create a family remedy chest (see p. 219).

Never leave herbs in plastic containers or plastic wrapping as this diminishes their shelf-life. You can store herbs in paper bags, but in this case you need extra care to safeguard them from damp and insects. Label the container with the name of the herb and the date, or you may forget which herbs are which, and how long you have been storing them.

Growing Herbs

If you want to buy an already-growing plant, check that the specimen comes from a good supplier and is healthy and free from pests. Plants that have been grown organically will be free from pesticide or herbicide residues, and will not have been grown with chemical fertilizers. This will ensure that only the most natural and healthy substances enter your body.

Dosages

Dosages for herbal remedies will depend on the method of preparation and the age of the person taking them. It is important to use just one system of measurement for dosages and recipes, so stick to metric or imperial throughout.

- Infusions and decoctions are taken in cupfuls or milliliters. Each cupful is approximately 8 fl oz (200 ml) and a potful is approximately 1¼ pints (600 ml).
- Tinctures are given in much smaller dosages due to their potency, usually teaspoons or drops. One teaspoon is 5 ml and one milliliter is about 20 drops.
- Medicinal wines are usually taken as one sherry glassful approximately 5 tbs (70 ml) a day.
- Syrups should be taken by the teaspoonful, usually between one and two teaspoons may be taken three times a day.

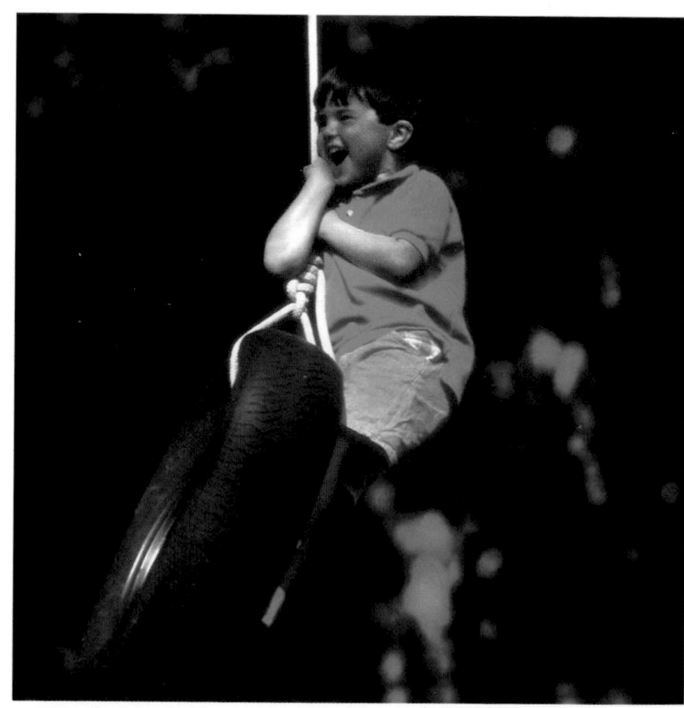

Right Children respond well to herbal remedies. Always check the correct dosage for each herb, based on the age of your child (see opposite).

Guidelines for dosages according to age

Babies to six months
Should only have herbal remedies under the guidance of an experienced herbal practitioner.

Babies six months to one year
One-tenth of an adult dose. If the mother is breastfeeding the baby will receive the correct amount if the mother takes the normal dosage. It is important to consult a qualified practitioner.

Children one to six years
One-third of the normal adult dose.

Children six to twelve years
One-half of the normal adult dose.

Adults
Infusions 3–4 cups* a day
Decoctions 2–3 cups a day
Tincture 1 tsp (5 ml) 2–3 times a day

Over 70s
Infusions 2–3 cups a day
Decoctions 1–2 cups a day
Tincture 1 tsp (5 ml) 2–3 times a day

**A cup is approximately 8 fl oz (200 ml)*

Pregnancy
Many herbs are useful in pregnancy, but it is advisable to check all remedies with a qualified practitioner before use.

Infusions

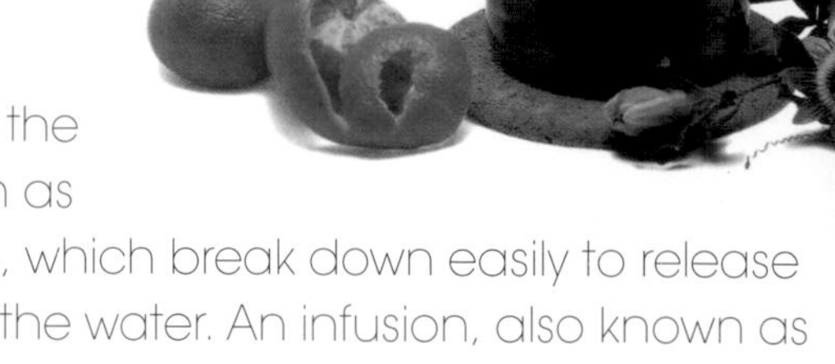

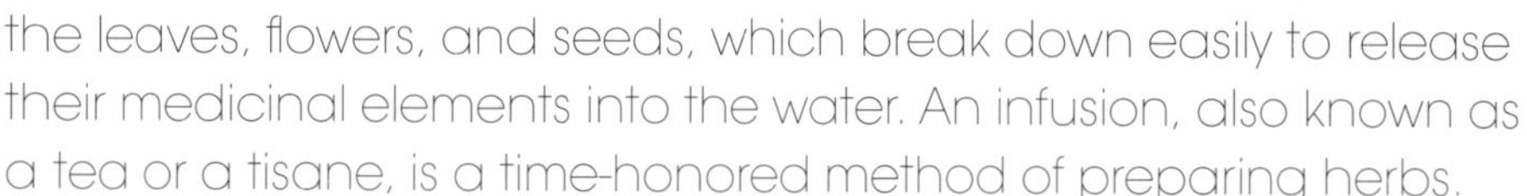

Infusions are used to prepare the delicate parts of a plant, such as the leaves, flowers, and seeds, which break down easily to release their medicinal elements into the water. An infusion, also known as a tea or a tisane, is a time-honored method of preparing herbs.

Above right When selecting appropriate herbs for your infusions choose one that adds a pleasant taste, such as lemon balm, so that your tea is refreshing as well as health-giving.

Making An Infusion

If making the infusion in a pot, do not use a pot used for making regular tea because the tannin will overpower the ingredients in the herbal tea. If you are making your tea in a teacup, you will need to cover it with a lid because some of the constituents of the tea include volatile oils, which evaporate in steam, and so the tea will lose much of its medicinal value if left uncovered. It may be kept for up to 24 hours in a refrigerator.

To prepare a pot of tea, warm the vessel and place the herbs in the pot. Add freshly boiled water. Replace the lid and leave to steep for 10 minutes. Using a tea strainer, pour the tea into a cup. To make a single cup, place the herbs in a tea-strainer on the cup and pour over freshly boiled water until it rises up and covers the herbs. Cover and leave for 10 minutes. Honey can be added if desired.

Cold and Flu Tea

½ yarrow
½ elderflower
pinch of peppermint

This cold and flu remedy, suitable for adults, will lower a fever; reduce nasal catarrh, and promote sweating to help cleanse and restore the system.

Method

Using a teapot *You will need about 1¼ pt (600 ml) of boiling water, and approximately 1 oz (20 g) of dried, or 1½ oz (30 g) of fresh herbs.*

This will make enough tea to have three or four cups in a day. You may use a single herb, or a selection of two or three of equal proportions, made up to the above amount.

Using a cup *Use approximately 1–2 tsp (2 g) of dried, or 2–3 tsp (3 g) of fresh, herbs per cup.*

Drink a cup two or three times a day, depending on what dose is appropriate (see pp.26–27).

Decoctions

A decoction is used to prepare the more resilient parts of a plant the bark, roots, rhizomes, and berries—where the constituents in the herb are more difficult to extract. Decoctions are always boiled for a minimum of 10 minutes.

Method

1 oz (20 g) of dried, or 2 oz (40 g) fresh, herbs to about 1½ pt (750 ml) of water.

Sections of root or bark should be chopped as finely as possible in order to allow the boiling water to extract the maximum from the plant. Place in a pan, cover with cold water, and bring to a boil. Cover the pan with a tight-fitting lid and simmer for 10 minutes. Allow the preparation to cool before straining, pressing out as much liquid from the residue as possible in order not to waste any of the valuable properties extracted.

If you wish to combine the properties of two herbs, for example a root and a flower or leaf, the leaf should be added at the end of the simmering period. The mixture should then be left, covered, for 10 minutes. It is possible to keep this mixture for the same period as a normal decoction because the liquid has been sterilized.

Stress and Anxiety Drink

valerian root decoction
skullcap infusion
verbena infusion

This remedy for adults is helpful during times of stress. It will lessen anxiety and provide a tonic for the nervous system.

Below Decoctions are made in larger quantities and last longer than infusions because the boiling process sterilizes the liquid.

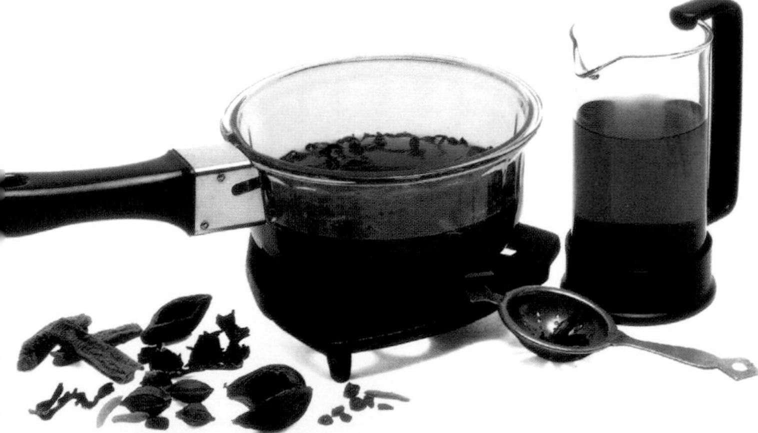

Tincture

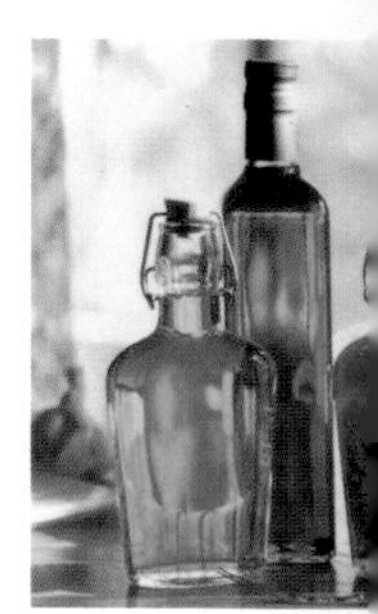

Tinctures can be used to prepare roots or leaves. They include alcohol and water to extract properties from the herbs which would not be available if a water preparation alone was used. It is possible to replace the alcohol with glycerol or vinegar.

Storage and Dosage

A tincture will last for up to two years and is a convenient method for the long-term use of the herbs. A tincture is much stronger than an infusion or a decoction, and is taken in teaspoons (tsp) or milliliters (ml) depending on the herb used. Use a dropper to measure amounts. In general, 20 drops = 1 ml. The average dose will vary between ⅕ tsp (1 ml) three times a day, and 1 tsp (5 ml) three times a day. Always check individual herbal dosages (see Herbal Directory pp.164–217) and label tinctures with the name of the herb and the date.

Tincture for Sleeplessness

4 oz (100 g) German camomile
½ pt (250 ml) vodka
1½ pt (750 ml) water

This tincture is excellent as an aid to restful sleep. Begin by taking 1 tsp (5 ml) approximately 20 minutes before going to bed. If this is not effective take a further 1 tsp (5 ml). You may take a maximum of 3 tsp (15 ml) in one night.

Method

The ratio of herb to liquid is one part herb to one part liquid. The liquid is made up of 25 per cent alcohol and 75 per cent water. You will need 8 oz (200 g) dried herb, ½ pt (250 ml) alcohol and 1½ pints (750 ml) water*

Finely chop the herbs and place them in a glass vessel or jar with a tightly fitting lid. Cover the herbs with the liquid and secure the lid. The jar should be placed in a warm, dark place for fourteen days. Shake the mixture every two or three days. At the end of this time, strain the mixture into a clean jar, keeping the remains of the wet herbs to one side. These can be pressed to extract every drop of the tincture by using a wine press, if you have one, or by wrapping the herbs in a muslin cloth and wringing out the last few drops. Keep the tincture in a colored glass jar or bottle, and store in a dark place.

**The alcohol should be at least 30 per cent proof in order to extract constituents and to preserve them. Suitable mediums include gin and vodka. Never use industrial alcohol. Always label tinctures with the name of the herb and the date.*

Medicinal Wines

Wines have long been used for medicinal purposes. There are two main ways to make a medicinal wine. The first is to use a commercially bought wine—preferably organic—and steep herbs in it. The second is to make the wine yourself.

Method 1

4 oz (100 g) dried herbs, 2 pints (1 liter) red or white wine

Place the herbs in a glass jar with a tight-fitting lid and cover with wine. Seal and leave to steep for at least two weeks. Filter and rebottle before use.

Iron Tonic Recipe (Method 1)

2 oz (40 g) dried nettle
2 oz (40 g) chopped apricots
2 pints (1 liter) red wine

This wine can be used as a tonic for anemic conditions where there is lethargy and tiredness, and also for dry eczema.

Method 2

1 whole root ginger, peeled, 2¼ lb (1 kg) sugar, rind and juice of 2 lemons and 2 oranges, 1 banana, good pinch cayenne pepper, 8 oz (200 g) raisins or golden raisins, yeast compound, 1 large pot of tea

This wine combines the qualities of ginger and cayenne. Squeeze the oranges and lemons, then slice the banana. Grate the ginger. Chop lemons and oranges, and add the raisins, cayenne pepper, and 1 lb (450 g) of sugar. Place in a demijohn. Make a large pot of regular tea and pour over the ingredients in the demijohn. Allow the sugar to dissolve and the mixture to cool slightly, then add a general-purpose yeast compound. Loosely stopper the demijohn. Leave to ferment for at least a week, adding tea until the demijohn is about two-thirds full. Then strain the fruit and ginger and return the strained liquid. Add the rest of the sugar and top up with tea if necessary. Continue to ferment for another week, then bottle.

Left Ginger is a warming, circulatory stimulant. It is excellent for colds as it is anti-inflammatory, antiseptic, and helps to soothe coughing. Cayenne is used as a remedy for sore throats and poor circulation.

Gargles and Mouthwashes

A gargle or mouthwash can be made from an infusion, a decoction, or a diluted tincture. It may be used for a variety of complaints associated with the mouth and throat. A gargle may help to soothe a sore and irritated throat associated with a cold or laryngitis.

Right A mouthwash or gargle made from an infusion, decoction, or diluted tincture (pp.28–30) can be used to keep breath fresh and to relieve tender gums or troublesome mouth ulcers.

Antiseptic Properties

Choose herbs that are known for their antiseptic properties. It is safe to swallow some of the liquid as you are gargling, bearing in mind the daily recommended dosage of the herb used and any general cautions (see Herbal Directory pp.164–215). A gargle may be used four or five times a day. Where there is persistent gum trouble, seek further help from your dentist or doctor to rule out any underlying problems. If mouth ulcers continually recur, this can suggest a problem which may need further treatment, and you should seek advice from a qualified practitioner.

Mouth Freshening Recipe

1 cup sage tea

A simple infusion of sage is ideal to relieve a sore throat, or simply to refresh the mouth. The volatile oils in sage help to cleanse and protect against bacteria, which can cause infection and damage teeth or gums.

Methods

Make an infusion of herb tea, allow to stand for 10 minutes, then leave to cool as required. Strain, and use as a gargle or mouthwash.

Tinctures

Dilute 1 tsp (5 ml) of the chosen tincture in 4 fl oz (100 ml) of water; and use as indicated on p.30.

Eyewashes

An eyewash or eyebath can be a refreshing way to relieve tired eyes caused by working for long periods under artificial lights and at computer screens. An eyewash can also relieve eye irritation caused by pollen or pollution.

Hygiene

To ensure no bacteria come into contact with the eyes, all utensils must be sterilized by boiling before use. If you have only one eyebath, treat one eye, then re-sterilize before bathing the other.

Preparing an Eyewash

The eyewash is prepared in the same way as an infusion, but first boil the water for 10 minutes before pouring it over the herbs. The liquid needs to be strained very carefully to avoid particles from the herbs being transferred to the eyes. Allow the liquid to cool before applying. If you are using eyebaths frequently, add a little salt to the bath to help rebalance the eye's natural fluid.

Using the Eyebath

Place the liquid in the eyebath and cover the eye, tipping the head back to allow the solution to gently bathe it. If any discomfort or irritation occurs stop treatment immediately. If an infected condition persists, seek advice from a qualified practitioner.

Conjunctivitis Remedy (Method 2)

½ cup eyebright tea
½ cup calendula tea

This remedy combines eyebright to reduce inflammation, and calendula for its antiseptic healing qualities.

Method 1

Make a compress by soaking a piece of cotton or lint in the eyebath infusion. Allow to cool, and place on the eyelids for 10–15 minutes.

Method 2

Prepare an infusion as described (see p.28). Leave to cool until lukewarm, then fill an eyebath and bathe the eyes. Twice a day should be sufficient.

Baths

Baths can be cleansing, relaxing, or revitalizing. When you add herbs to your bath, you can enhance the benefits of your usual bathtime routine. Either infusions or decoctions can be used in baths or you may wish to try the benefits of essential oils.

Whole-Body Bath

Add 1¼ pt (600 ml) herbal infusion to your normal bath water. Mix well. Alternatively, add roughly five drops essential oils to the bath while the water is running*. Try an infusion of lavender to relax in the evening, rosemary to invigorate in the morning, and thyme to soothe aching muscles. Do not allow the bath to get too cold or the benefits will be lost.

Hand Bath

Using a suitable bowl or basin, immerse the whole hand up to the wrist in the cooled, strained herbal infusion. Make sure your position is comfortable: allow it to rest in a relaxed manner. For hot, painful arthritic joints, use a cooling infusion such as peppermint, for a cold, aching joint, a hotter infusion of ginger is warming. Immersion should last between 5 and 10 minutes. Finally, make sure you dry your hands thoroughly afterward.

Below If a whole-body bath is not possible, for example, in cases of illness or infirmity, a hand or foot bath can provide relief.

Foot Bath

This is especially good for relaxing tired, aching feet at the end of a long day. One of the simplest remedies for a cold is to sit with your feet in a bowl of fairly hot water and add a heaped teaspoon of mustard powder. Sit for 10 minutes, then dry your feet.

Body Wash

Prepare an infusion of your chosen herb, strain, and, using a clean cloth, gently bathe the selected area. Tepid water is best for this type of wash. Dry gently.

**Do not use essential oils in baby baths as babies can ingest oils through mouth/hand contact.*

Inhalations

A steam inhalation can be used to relieve conditions such as colds, flu, catarrh, and sinusitus. The steam helps to relax the airways, and ease mucus membranes.

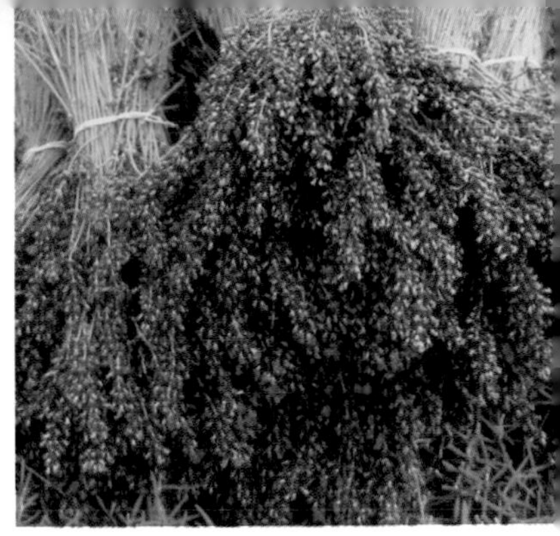

Above The addition of an herbal remedy, such as lavender, to a steam inhalation helps to ease congestion and for young children a steamy bathroom can be beneficial for colds.

Method

Approximately 2 pints (1 liter) of liquid is needed. Prepare an infusion of your chosen herb by adding freshly boiled water, then pour immediately into a bowl ready for use. (It is best to take the infusion to the bowl rather than carrying a heavy, rather hot, bowl from room to room.) If using essential oils, first boil the water and pour into the bowl, then add between three to six drops of the oil to the liquid and stir. Sit comfortably and place a large towel or cloth over your head and the bowl so that no steam escapes. Continue this treatment for about 10 minutes or until the water cools, but do come up for air if you need to. Afterward, sit in a warmed room for about half an hour to allow your respiratory system to adjust to the outside temperature.

Vaporizers

If you wish to use a less-concentrated inhalation, an oil vaporizer (sometimes called a diffuser) placed in a room is ideal. Vaporizers come in many different designs and shapes. Generally, they consist of a small nightlight candle with a bowl above, into which the water and essential oil are poured. It is important to fill the bowl. A half-filled bowl may crack because the light will continue to burn after the water has evaporated. Use between one and six drops of essential oil. If a vaporizer is not available, essential oil added to a bowl filled with boiling water will allow the vapor to diffuse throughout the room. Or a drop or two of oil on a piece of cotton or clean cloth placed above a radiator* will have much the same effect.

Tension Recipe

3–5 drops lavender essential oil
bowl of hot water/diffuser

Lavender has a calming, sedative effect. If tension prevents you from winding down after a hard day, add a lavender infusion to a bowl of water or a diffuser, and allow your cares to drift away.

**Never place items directly onto a radiator or where any part of it touches the radiator.*

Infused Oils and Ointments

Infused oils can be used for massage or as a base oil to which essential oils can be added. They can also be used as the base for preparing ointments. These are oil-based preparations which form a protective layer on the skin to aid the healing process.

Which Oils to Use

Infused oils are different from essential oils and can be made easily and cheaply at home. The best oils for infusions are vegetable, either sunflower or soya. There are two ways of making an infused oil: a cold preparation where the oils are heated by the sun, and a hot preparation where the oils are heated gently on the stove. Always handle hot oils carefully and never use them internally or allow them to come into contact with the eyes. Oils will last for about a year.

Nerve Tonic Oil

St. John's wort flowers
vegetable oil

The flowers of St. John's wort are yellow, but as the plant oils are diffused into the vegetable oil, the color will turn deep red. This oil is excellent for gently massaging into areas where there is nerve strain or pain, for example, in cases of repetitive strain injury or neuralgia.

Method

4 oz (100 g) dried herb or 8 oz (200 g) fresh herb, 16 fl oz (400 ml) vegetable oil

Cold Oils This method is very easy but slow. Use a clean, dry jar with a tight-fitting lid and pack it full with your chosen herb. Pour the oil into the jar, covering the herbs completely. Put the lid on and place it on a warm, sunny windowsill for about two weeks, shaking and turning the jar daily. After two weeks strain the oil carefully, using a muslin bag or cloth stretched over a bowl. Make sure all plant material is removed, and squeeze every last drop of oil to get the maximum benefit. Store oils in dark bottles away from sunlight. Do not forget to label and date your preparation.

Hot Oils This process is more complicated, using a double boiler—a pan filled with water, brought to a boil and gently simmering, over which a larger pan or glass bowl is placed—but it produces a good-

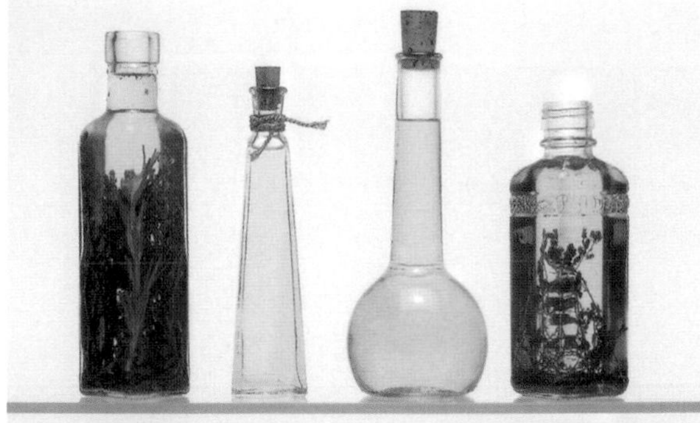

Above Hot and cold oil infusions can be used for massage and also as a base when making creams and ointments.

quality oil. The vegetable oil and herb are put into the double boiler, so the oil never comes into direct contact with the heat. Cover the pan or bowl containing the oil and herb with a tight-fitting lid. Leave for a minimum of two hours, and allow to cool before filtering the oil into a clean bowl, using a cloth or straining bag. Repeat the double boiling but using fresh herbs to give double strength to your oil. Strain the oil and discard the herbs. Bottle your oil in dark glass jars, and store away from sunlight.

Ointments for Sensitive Skin

Homemade herbal creams and ointments are ideal for those with sensitive or allergic skin because you can choose your own ingredients and minimize the use of additives or preservatives, which can cause irritation. Ointments are suited for use where areas of skin are exposed to the elements, for example chapped lips or dry eczema. Before using any remedy on the skin first try a patch test. Apply a little of the ointment or cream on to an area of skin and leave it for 24 hours. If any reaction occurs, discontinue use. Seek medical advice if the irritation persists.

Method

8 fl oz (200 ml) infused oil, 1 oz (20 g) beeswax (grated), 2–5 drops essential oil

Fill a pan with water, bring to a boil and then reduce to a simmer. Place another pan or glass bowl over the boiling water and pour in the oil. Add grated beeswax gradually, stirring until the wax is melted before adding any essential oils you wish to use. Remove the bowl from the heat, and carefully pour into a clean glass jar and allow to set. Seal the jar, then label and date it.

Ointment for Cuts and Scrapes

8 fl oz (200 ml) infused calendula oil
1 oz (20 g) beeswax
2 drops lavender essential oil

This ointment combines the anti-bacterial properties of calendula with the astringent and anti-inflammatory qualities of lavender.

Creams

Skin creams combine oil and a water-based medium to create a mixture which nourishes and enriches the skin. Creams that are firm act as a barrier against the elements, while those of liquid consistency can be used to cleanse and moisturize.

Soothing Cream
7 tsp (75 ml) chickweed infusion
2 tsp (10 ml) oil
1 tsp (5 ml) emulsifying wax
3 drops camomile essential oil
Chickweed is extremely cooling and is an effective relief for itching. Camomile essential oil combines anti-allergenic and anti-inflammatory properties.

Preparing a Cream

Creams are more difficult to prepare than ointments since the oil and water base must be carefully blended or the two ingredients will separate out. The water base portion of the recipe can be either an infusion or a decoction of the chosen herbs. An agent is required to facilitate the blending process, usually emulsifying wax.

How Much to Make

Because a cream includes water, its shelflife will be less than an ointment, therefore prepare only a small quantity. To preserve and enhance the quality of the cream it is possible to add an essential oil. A cream should always be stored in a cool place or in the refrigerator.

Method

7 parts infusion/decoction, 2 parts oil, 1 part emulsifying wax

If you are using teaspoons, the recipe will use seven teaspoons of infusion, two teaspoons of oil, and one teaspoon of emulsifying wax. Mix in three drops of essential oil to each 1½ oz (30 g) jar made. Fill a pan with water, bring to the boil, and simmer. Place a second pan or bowl over the first and pour in the oil and infusion. Gradually add the emulsifying wax, stirring until it is dissolved. Remove the bowl from the heat, and place it in a bowl filled with cold water. It is important to keep stirring the mixture as it cools or the ingredients will separate. Add the essential oil and mix well. Spoon the mixture into glass jars, replace the lids, label, and date. Store in the refrigerator.

Syrups

Syrups are soothing mixtures which are popular with adults and children alike. You can turn an infusion, a decoction, or a tincture into a syrup by combining the liquid-based remedy with sugar or honey. This will also improve the taste of less-pleasant herbs.

Method

8 fl oz (200 ml) infusion, 8 oz (200 g) sugar/honey

Infusion-based Syrup For this type of syrup, you will need equal amounts of infusion and sugar. Prepare your infusion in the usual manner, but leave it to steep for 15 rather than 10 minutes.

Strain the tea as usual through a cloth, taking care to press out as much of the liquid as possible. The liquid should then be heated gently in a pan and the sugar or honey added. Stir constantly to dissolve all the sugar, taking care not to boil the mixture.

Allow the syrup to cool, then carefully pour into bottles, seal, and label. Store in a cool, dark place. (Take care, when sealing, that the lid is left slightly loose as tightly stoppered bottles have been known to explode after a time.)

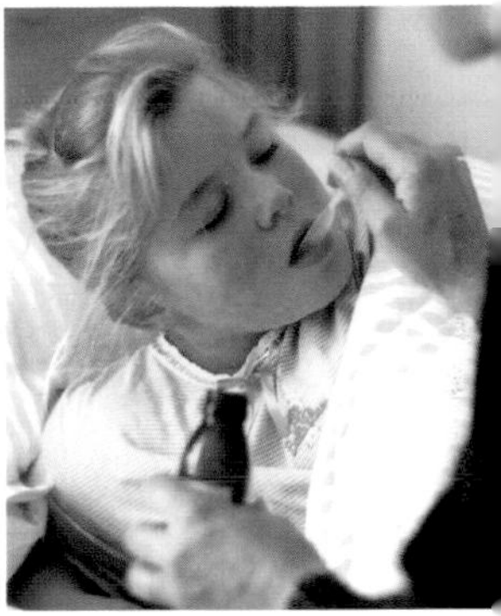

Above Syrups are sweet and easily swallowed and so they are useful in the treatment of coughs and sore throats, especially for children.

Decoction-based Syrup This method is exactly the same as for infusion-based syrups except that the decoction should be simmered for 30 minutes.

Tincture-based Syrup

4 fl oz (100 ml) water, 8 oz (200 g) sugar, 4 fl oz (100 ml) tincture

First prepare the syrup, and then add the tincture. Boil the water, and then add it to the sugar or honey, which are in another pan. Stir until all the sugar is dissolved, then remove from the heat. Allow to cool, then stir in the tincture. Bottle, seal, and label as before. The quantities used are always the same ratio, that is, one-part tincture to three-parts syrup.

Recipe for Cough Syrup

8 fl oz (200 ml) infusion of thyme
8 oz (200 g) unrefined sugar

This remedy uses the antiseptic and expectorant qualities of thyme to relieve coughs and sore throats.

Vinegars

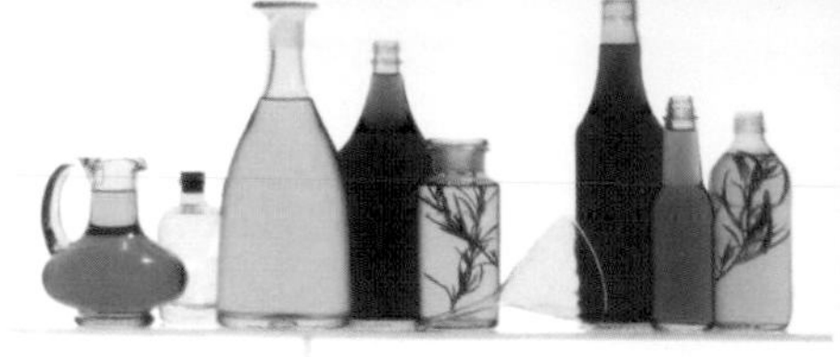

Vinegars can be used in a similar way to tinctures, and can provide an alternative for those who do not find either the alcoholic or glycerine preparations suitable. Vinegar contains acetic acid, which helps to preserve and extract the essential ingredients of herbs.

Above In addition to their medicinal function, vinegars are an interesting way to complement foods. Apple cider or wine vinegars, preferably organic, are the most versatile.

Preparation

Use a jar or bottle with a wide mouth. Choose your herb, making sure it is as dry as possible. Place the herb in the jar and top up with the vinegar. Store for a minimum of two weeks (some sources recommend one or two months) in a dark place, shaking every day. Then strain off the liquid and bottle. The vinegar should be left for a further two weeks before using.

Dosage

Herb vinegars can be taken internally in the same way as tinctures, that is, by the teaspoonful, or added to salads, soups, or as an ingredient in pickles. Externally they can be added to bathwater, and used as a lotion, or even a hair rinse. The recipes given below show how versatile vinegars can be.

Itchy-Skin Lotion

Elderflower blossoms, apple cider vinegar

The flowers of the elder tree are noted for their anti-inflammatory action. Especially valued for internal use in allergic conditions, the flowers can also be used in a vinegar base as an external wash to calm and soothe itching skin, especially in cases of allergic reactions. It can also be used to alleviate the painful burning of an insect sting.

Dry-Scalp Rinse

Nettle tops, white wine vinegar

The astringent properties of nettle and the softening effects of vinegar combine to help bring a shine to dull hair and encourage circulation to a dry scalp. Add a little of the vinegar to your final rinsing water.

Poultices and Compresses

Traditionally, poultices are used to draw out toxins from the body, promote circulation, and aid healing. Poultices and compresses are applied in the same way, but are prepared differently and perform different functions.

Fresh Herb Poultice

First, apply a little sunflower or vegetable oil to the skin to prevent sticking. Crush the plant and then place it directly on to the affected area. Hold the poultice in place with a dressing or bandage.

Dried Herb Poultice

Dried herbs must first be decocted by simmering them in a pan of water for approximately five minutes. Allow the mixture to cool. Squeeze out the liquid and keep the remaining material. Place the herbs on to a dressing, and spread evenly. Apply to the affected area.

Cooling Compress

8 fl oz (200 ml) lavender infusion

A lavender compress can be placed on the forehead or the back of the neck to relieve tension and headaches. Soak a clean face cloth in the infusion and wring it out. Wrap the damp cloth in plastic wrap and place in the refrigerator for at least two hours before use.

Powdered Herb Poultice

First mix the powders with a cold liquid, either water or a tincture. Stir until you get a fine paste, then spread on a bandage as above.

Compresses

Compresses are applied directly to the skin, but in this case it is the liquid from the mixture that is used. A compress can utilize either an infusion, a decoction, or a tincture. If using a tincture, it should be diluted with a little water. You will need a clean cloth for soaking in the liquid. Once the liquid portion is prepared, the cloth should be soaked thoroughly and then wrung out. To retain moisture, cover with plastic wrap or a plastic bag, and secure with a bandage. Replace as needed.

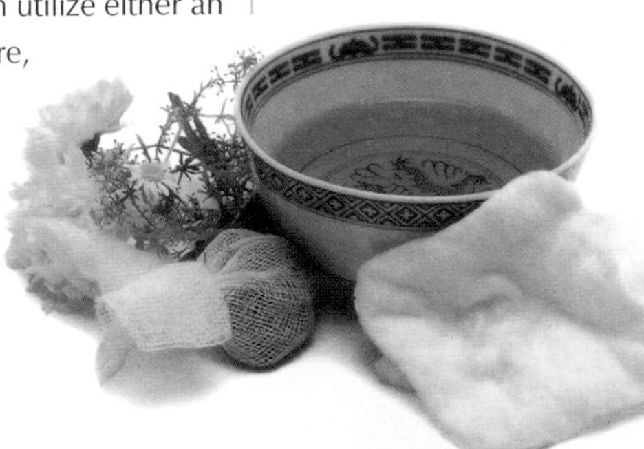

Below Use a cool poultice or compress for hot, inflamed conditions and a warm application to relieve aches and strains.

Chinese Herbal Decoctions

The word for decoction, "tang", literally means "soup". It is one of the most common ways of taking a combination of traditional Chinese herbs. Use the guidelines below to make your own decoctions.

Below Several Chinese herbs mentioned in this book need to be prepared differently. The volatile oils, which give these herbs their fragrance, are part of their healing qualities but they can easily be destroyed by over-cooking.

Quantities

Use approximately 1½ pints (800 ml) water with 1½ oz (30 g) of Chinese herbs. The common dosage is ⅛–½ oz (3–10 g) per herb daily, but be sure to take note of the dosages recommended for individual herbs in the Herbal Directory (pp.164–215). Children, the elderly, pregnant women, and anyone with a weak digestive system must take them in smaller dosages. If a traditional Chinese herbalist includes many herbs in a prescription, a daily dosage of 3–4½ oz (80–120 g) may be given.

Preparation

There are a variety of ways of preparing a decoction, depending on the herbs used and the practitioner prescribing them. Always use a non-aluminum pot. Soak the herbs for two hours. Tonic herbs, such as astragalus (*huang qi*), Chinese angelica (*dang gui*), and licorice (*gan cao*), which are used to strengthen the system, should be simmered gently in a covered pot for one hour. Herbs for more acute conditions, such as chrysanthemum (*ju hua*), burdock (*nui bang zi*), dandelion (*pu gong ying*), and honeysuckle (*jin yin hua*), should be simmered for 20–30 minutes. Strain the herbs from the liquid and drink warm, in equal doses, morning and evening. Peppermint (*bo he*) and perilla leaf (*zi su ye*) should be added in the last five minutes of preparation.

Ginseng

A piece of good ginseng root is valued highly in China for its life-enhancing properties. Put 1⁄16–½ oz (1–9 g) ginseng in a small amount of water placed over a double boiler. Simmer for an hour, then strain off the liquid. Add this to liquid from other herbal decoctions, or drink it on its own. The ginseng root can be cooked in this way several times to extract all the goodness and to use it efficiently.

Chinese Patent Formulas

Chinese patent formulas are classical herbal prescriptions that can be taken in pill or tincture form and are freely available. These traditional formulas can be effective for a wide range of ailments.

Traditional Chinese patent formulas are still imported from China by most suppliers of Chinese herbs and are available online as well as in stores. Many Western manufacturers have adapted the traditional formulas to treat modern Western conditions. The Western adaptations often list the traditional formula on which the prescription is based, which is a handy reference to some of the more commonly available prescriptions.

The Chinese Court

The classical Chinese herbal formulas, which have been used for many centuries, were often based on members of the Chinese court. These formulas consist of many herbs which work in balance and harmony. The Four Gentlemen Decoction (*Si Jun Zi Tang*), was derived from the Confucian term meaning an exemplary person, and the number four, whose nature is harmonious. The chief herb, also known as the emperor, or *jun* herb, is ginseng, which strengthens the *qi*, or energy, of the body. The minister, or *chen* herb, white atractylodis rhizome (*bai zhu*), acts as the advisor, and works synergistically. The assistant, or *zuo* herb, is poria (*fu ling*), which works to balance the cloying nature of the tonic herbs to make them more digestible. The envoy *shi* herb, honey-fried licorice (*zhi gan cao*), delivers the whole prescription to the digestive system and the twelve main channels of the body.

Women's Precious Pills (*Ba Zhen Wan*)

This is an excellent women's tonic which combines the two classical formulas: the Four Gentlemen, which strengthens the *qi*, or energy, and the Four Substances, which nourishes the blood. It is useful in conditions of tiredness, dizziness, irregular menstruation, scanty periods, poor circulation, and in the recovery from childbirth or long-term illness. It contains the herbs listed in the Four Gentlemen Decoction and Chinese angelica (*clang gui*), which is one of the herbs in the Four Substances which strengthens the blood and improves circulation. Take five pills, two to three times a day.

Nose Inflammation Pills (*Bi Yan Pian*)

A useful formula for symptoms related to allergies such as sneezing, itching eyes, and congested sinuses; it is also an excellent remedy for relieving symptoms of hayfever. It contains chrysanthemum flower (*ju hua*) and forsythia (*lian qiao*), which help to clear the first signs of colds. Take four tablets, three times a day, an hour after eating.

Central Qi Pills (*Bu Zhong Yi Qi Wan*)

A useful formula helping to strengthen and invigorate the digestion. It relieves symptoms of bloating, pain, wind, and alternating constipation and diarrhea. Also helps to raise the *yang*, or lift prolapses of the uterus and rectum, hemorrhoids, and varicose veins. It contains the Chinese herbs codonopsis root (*dang shen*)—which is a less-expensive substitute for ginseng—astragalus (*huang qi*), angelica (*dang gui*), and licorice (g*an cao*), all of which help support the immune system. These herbs also help to strengthen the digestion, along with citrus peel (*chen pi*), and ginger (*sheng jiang*), which aid movement of food through the system. Take five pills, two to three times a day.

Decoction For Frigid Extremities (*Dang Gui Si Ni Tang*)

Used to warm the extremities and nourish the blood, this formula is often taken in tincture form because it is easily absorbed into the bloodstream. It is useful in conditions of poor circulation, rheumatoid arthritis with cold symptoms, Raynaud's disease, and frostbite. It contains Chinese angelica (*dang gui*), which strengthens the blood and improves the circulation, and cinnamon (*gui zhi*), which is warming. It should be used with caution in the spring and summer, in warm climates, or with symptoms of heat, such as fever and sweating. Take one teaspoonful in warm water, three times a day.

Angelica and Loranthus Pill (*Du Huo Ji Sheng Wan*)

A formula used to strengthen the back and lower extremities and ease stiffness. It is helpful with low back pain, sciatica, and arthritis, especially when the condition is helped by heat and warmth, or due to deficiency. It contains Chinese angelica (*dang gui*), which encourages circulation, and the warming herbs of ginger (*sheng jiang*), and the inner bark of the cinnamon tree (*rou gui*). Take five pills, two to three times a day.

Ear-ringing Left Loving Pills (*Er Long Zuo Ci Wan*)

A variation of *Liu Wei Di Huang Wan* (see below), these pills help to ease symptoms of tinnitus, headache, high blood pressure, insomnia, thirst, and eye pressure and irritation. Take five pills, three times a day; they can be taken over a period of time.

Six-Flavor Rehmannia Pill (*Liu Wei Di Huang Wan*)

A classic Chinese herbal prescription, which forms the basis for other prescriptions. It is nourishing for the *yin* aspect, strengthening the liver, kidney, and spleen. It helps to ease symptoms of weakness or pain in the lower back, burning in the palms or soles of the feet, mild night sweats, dizziness, tinnitus, and a mild, constant sore throat. It can help high blood pressure and diabetes, but professional advice should first be sought. Take five pills, three times a day. These may be taken over a period of time, but may aggravate catarrhal conditions.

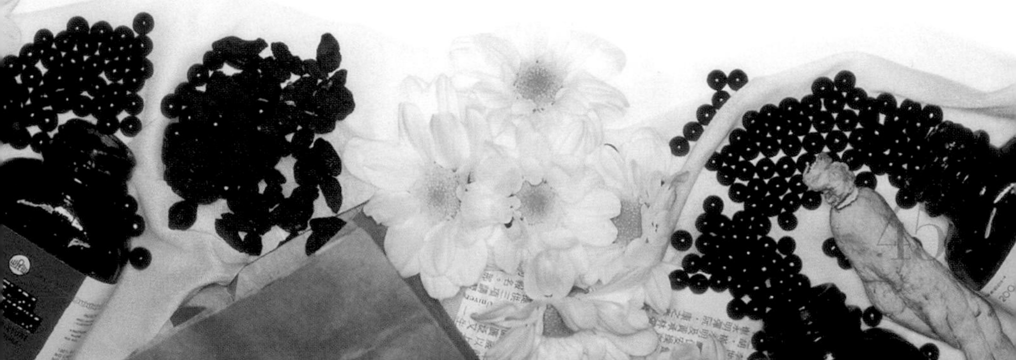

Below Chinese herbal patent remedies, based on traditional Chinese formulas, are a simple way of taking herbal treatments.

Bright Eyes Rehmannia Pills (*Ming Mu Di Huang Wan*)

Another variation of *Liu Wei Di Huang Wan* (see p.45) which helps to benefit many eye complaints especially in the elderly. This formula contains Chinese angelica (*dang gui*), which helps to nourish the blood and improve circulation. The herbs chrysanthemum flower (*ju hua*) and lycium fruit (*gou qi zi*) are particularly beneficial for the eyes. Take five pills, three times a day.

Lycium, Chrysanthemum, Rehmannia Pills (*Qi Ju Di Huang Wan*)

A variation of *Liu Wei Di Huang Wan* (see p.45) which helps to treat blurry vision, poor night vision, dry and painful eyes, and pressure behind the eyes. It differs from *Ming Mu Di Huang Wan* (see above) in that it also treats headache, dizziness, irritability, restlessness, and insomnia. It can be helpful with menopausal symptoms. As stated in its English name, this formula contains lycium fruit (*gou qi zi*) and chrysanthemum flower (*ju hua*), which help to nourish the eyes. Take five pills, three times a day.

Clean Air Tea (*Qing Qi Hua Tan Wan*)

A useful prescription for the treatment of asthma, chronic bronchitis, or sinus infection when there is a thick, sticky phlegm that is difficult to clear. Take five pills, three times a day.

Morus, Chrysanthemum Medicine Pill (*Sang Ju Yin Pian*)

A useful pill to clear the first signs of a cough, especially a dry one, accompanied by a dry, sore throat, sneezing, runny nose, and watery eyes. It contains forsythia fruit (*lian qiao*), chrysanthemum flower (*ju hua*), and peppermint (*bo he*), all of which help to eliminate symptoms of colds and flu. Take three tablets, two to three times a day.

Codonopsis, Poria, Atractylodes Formula (*Shen Ling Bai Zhu Pian*)

A useful formula for strengthening weak digestion. It helps to clear symptoms of bloating, indigestion, and loose stools. It is a good tonic for children with poor appetites and slow growth. Take five pills, three times a day. Children can take three pills, two to three times a day.

Zizyphus Seed Soup Tablet (*Suan Zao Ren Tang Pian*)

A prescription to calm the *shen* or "spirit of the heart," helping with problems of insomnia, restlessness, heart palpitations, and mental agitation. Take two tablets, three times a day.

Heavenly King Benefit Heart Pill (*Tian Wang Bu Xin Wan*)

Useful to calm the *shen* in cases where there is a deficiency or chronic tiredness. It is helpful with insomnia, anxiety, palpitations, and vivid dreaming. It is also used in treating hyperactive thyroid. Take five pills, three times a day.

Free and Easy Wanderer (*Xiao Yao Wan*)

A basic formula used to nourish the blood, move the *qi*, or energy, and strengthen the digestion. It is helpful for a range of symptoms, such as bloating and fullness in the abdomen, menstrual disorders, and tension headaches. The formula contains Chinese angelica (*dang gui*), which is useful for many menstrual problems. Take five pills, three times a day.

Lonicera, Forsythia Dispel Heat Tablets (*Yin Qiao Jie Du Pian*)

An excellent remedy to clear colds when taken with the first symptoms such as a sore throat, fever with chills, stiff muscles, and sneezing. This formula contains the following herbs used to dispel early symptoms of colds: peppermint (*bo he*), forsythia fruit (*lian qiao*), honeysuckle (*jin yin hua*), and burdock seed (*nui bang zi*). Take five pills, every three hours for the first nine hours, then every five hours as needed. Discontinue after three days.

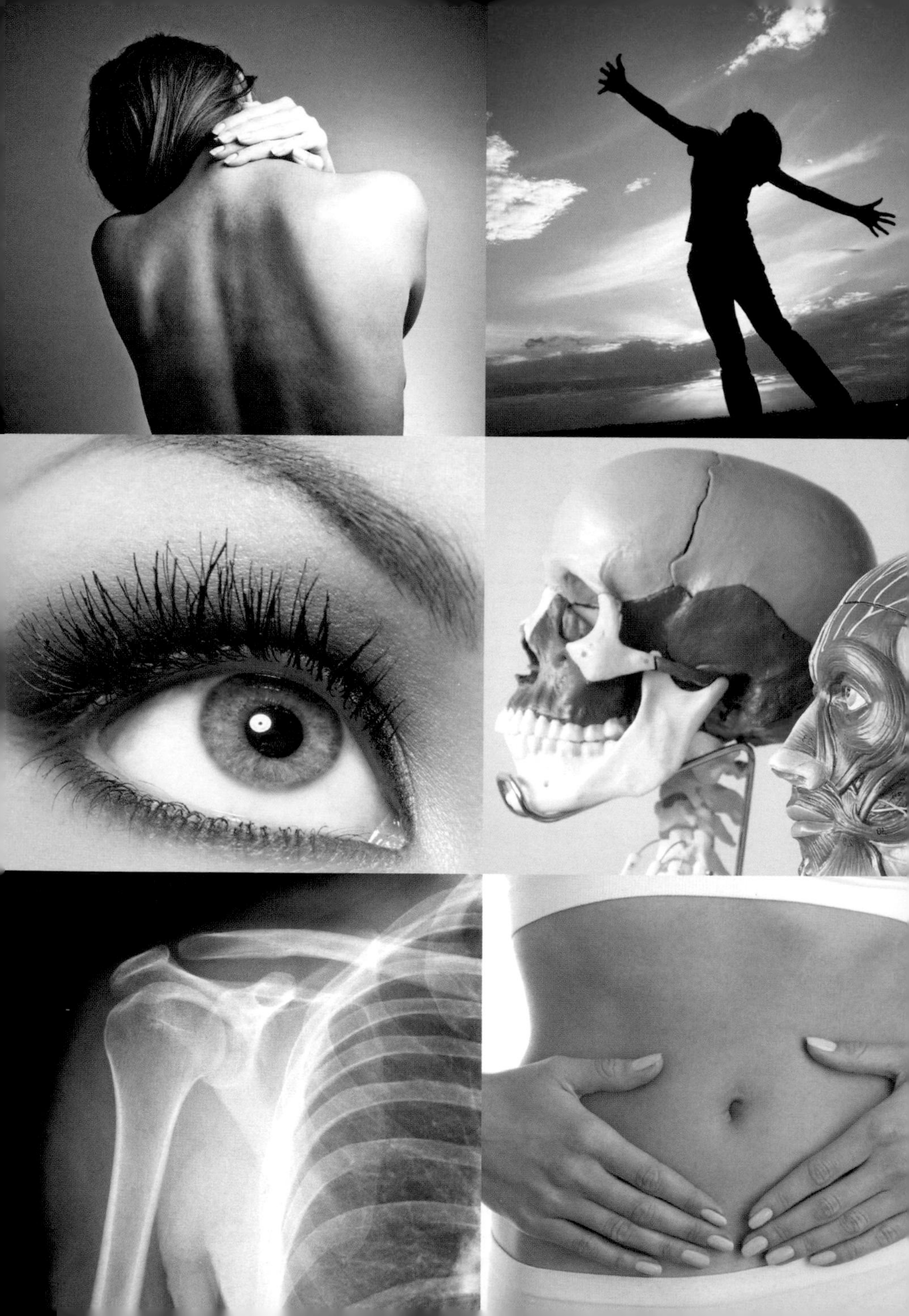

The Body

& How to Treat It

This section describes the different systems of the body and their related ailments. Herbal treatments and methods of application are suggested so that common complaints can be treated gently but effectively.

Healing Herbs

The ability to heal ourselves, to restore and revitalize our life force, or *qi*, lies within us. Plants offer simple remedies to help enhance our own healing process. Understanding how our body works helps us to appreciate its efficiency and ability to repair itself. We need to work with our body, not against it. Herbal medicine can help to support us so that we can bring about a deeper, permanent change within ourselves.

This section describes the different systems in the body and their related ailments. Within each system there is a brief description of how it works, its interaction to the rest of the body, and how it is viewed in terms of Chinese medicine. Suggestions for preventing illnesses and complaints are also given, including changes in diet, lifestyle, and outlook on life. Understanding the whole picture of your particular ailment will help the herbal healing process.

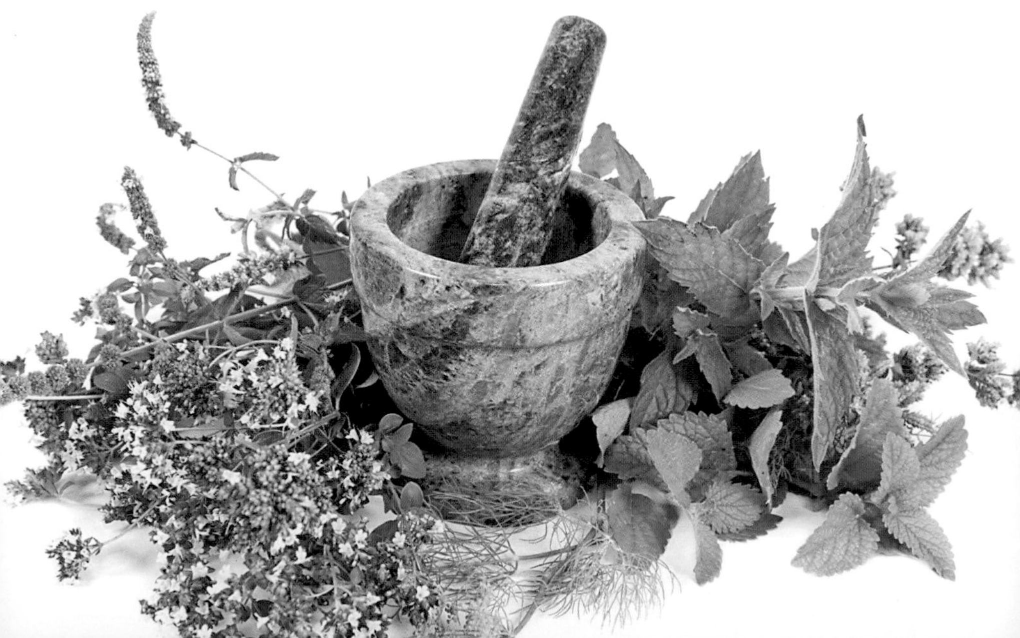

Choosing the Right Herbs for the Right Treatment

With most ailments, several suggestions for herbal treatment will be given. These will include combinations of herbs, Chinese remedies, and external herbal treatments.

Before using any herbs, please check the Herbal Directory (pp.164–215) to find out more about the herb, and be sure to note any cautions, contraindications, and dosages. Then read the Herbal Methods chapter (pp.20–47) to find out the most beneficial way of preparing the herb. If the specific dosages have not been given in the Herbal Directory (pp.164–215), use the recommended dosages listed on p.27. Be sure to take into account any changes in dosage given for both the elderly and children.

Cautions and Contraindications

Herbs are safe to use if taken in the right amount, with cautions and contraindications observed. There is much debate about herbal safety, and we have listed precautions we have found while researching this book. Pregnancy is one condition where care needs to be taken when using herbs. Digestive problems, skin complaints, and blood pressure may be aggravated with the use of certain herbs, so please check the Herbal Directory (pp.164–215) beforehand. Care must also be taken with essential oils; they should not be taken internally or used for babies. Please read the Herbal Directory carefully, and seek advice from a professional herbalist if you have any doubts about the use of a herb.

Combining Herbs and Drugs

If you are taking medication for a serious medical problem, it is best to seek advice from a professional medical herbalist and your doctor. Herbs can be used with most medications, but it is important to select the most appropriate ones. DO NOT STOP TAKING ANY MEDICATION without the advice of your doctor and herbalist. Be aware that taking herbs may change your need for medication, and this must be monitored regularly.

Opposite A balanced diet, regular physical exercise, and a positive attitude help to keep us healthy. Herbal medicine supports our natural flow of energy helping to gently heal us.

When Herbs are Ineffective

Herbal treatment will vary with different types of conditions. Acute infections, such as colds and flu, will need a treatment that has an immediate effect, while more chronic conditions, such as arthritis, will need long-term treatment. Generally, you will know in a matter of days whether an acute infection is clearing, as the symptoms will become better quickly. If one herb does not work, try some of the other herbs mentioned. If no herbal treatments seem to be effective, it is probably time to call a doctor, as symptoms of acute infections such as fever, vomiting, or diarrhea can be debilitating and dangerous if left for more than a few days. With chronic conditions it is sometimes hard to know if the herbs are helping as the symptoms may vary from day to day. Herbal treatment may need to take place over a period of several weeks, and diet and lifestyle may also require changes. If the condition generally has not improved after several weeks, you may need to consult a professional herbalist to find the right herbs.

Home Care and Professional Herbalism

Most of the herbal suggestions in this book are safe to use as a way of looking after ourselves, our families, and friends. Herbal baths, vaporizers, and simple herbal teas can be used as part of a daily routine that helps maintain good health and feelings of well-being. There may be times when you need professional advice from an herbalist as the condition is too serious to be treated without experience and training. Make sure that you go to an herbalist who is registered with a recognized professional body or institute. The herbalist will take a case history and prescribe appropriate herbs; they will also be supportive in helping you to make any other changes needed.

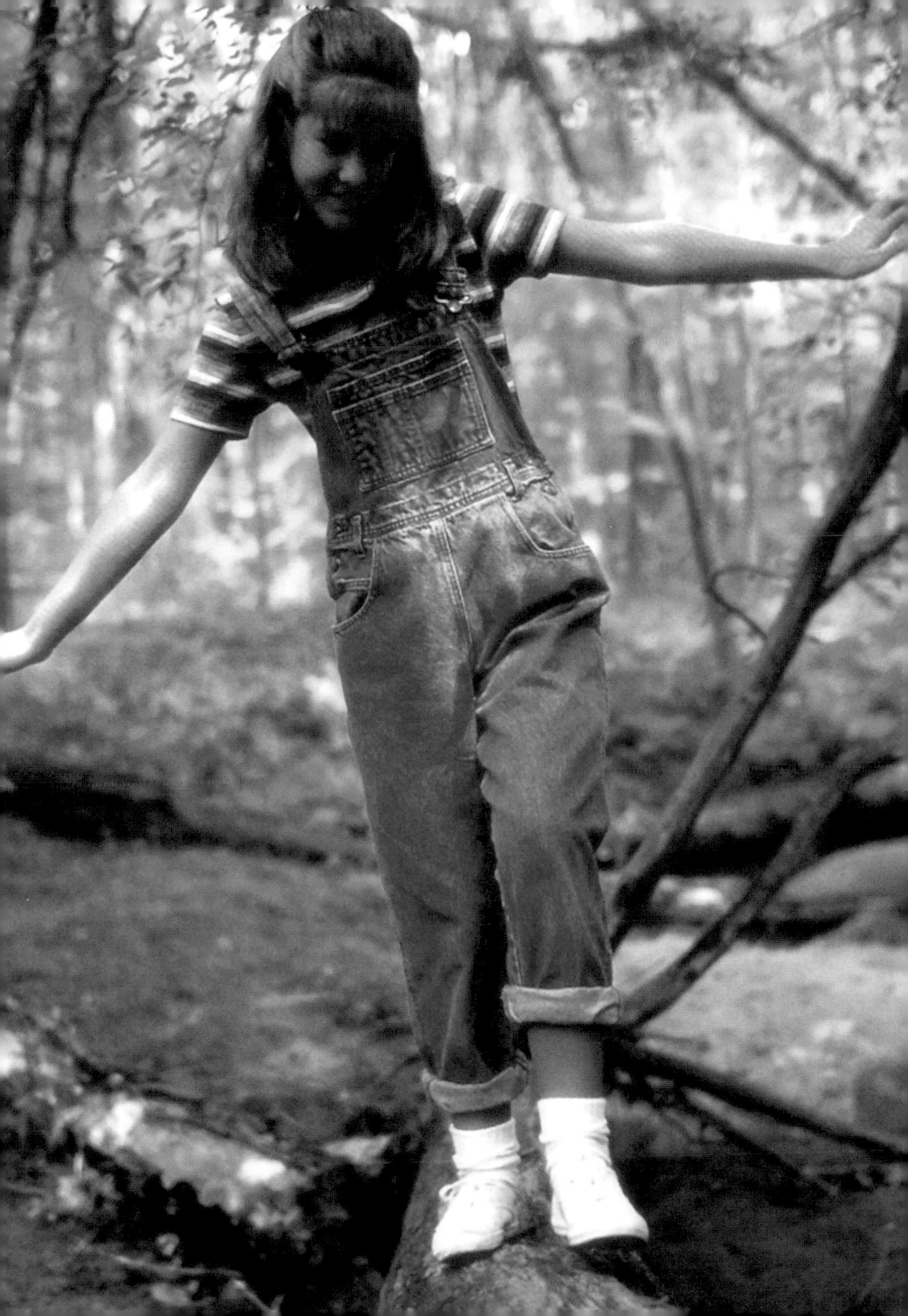

Respiration

We can only survive a matter of minutes without breathing. The air we breathe brings us the essential element which is vital for life: oxygen. Our respiratory system needs to be in good working order to take in revitalizing oxygen, and filter out the toxins that are now so much a part of our environment.

Our first contact with air is through the nose and mouth. Our nose alerts us to the smell of the air—is it fresh and fragrant, or full of toxic fumes? Sometimes we can even taste the poisonous gases in the air, and our reaction may be to hold our breath for several seconds. Infectious bacteria from someone who is ill also pass through the air. Our nose, mouth, and throat are our first line of defense. They contain cilia, or tiny hairs, that cleanse the nose and throat by pulling mucus and saliva into the stomach, where it is sterilized. Saliva and mucus protect the delicate lining of the mouth and nose by trapping invasive particles. Under healthy conditions these mechanisms work very well to keep us free from illness.

Right Our sense of smell allows us to enjoy pleasant scents, but our nose also helps to defend us from infection.

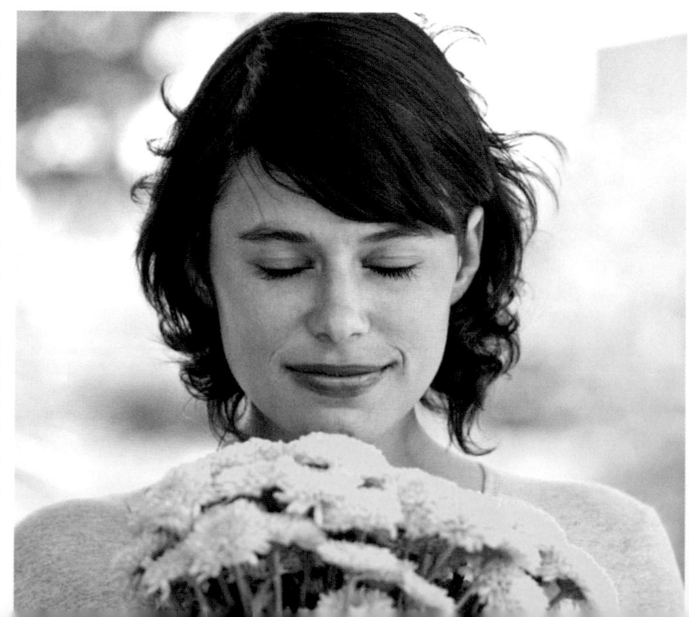

How Respiration Works

The respiratory system is responsible for introducing oxygen into the blood, which carries it to the tissues, and for removing carbon dioxide from the blood.

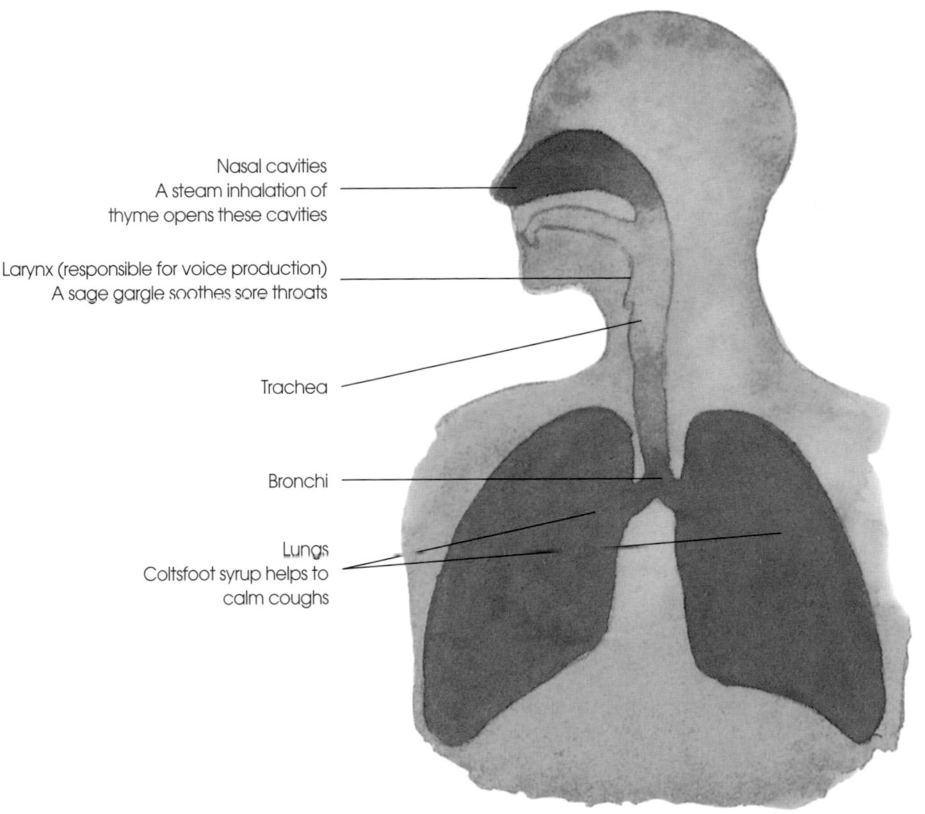
Nasal cavities
A steam inhalation of
thyme opens these cavities
Larynx (responsible for voice production)
A sage gargle soothes sore throats
Trachea
Bronchi
Lungs
Coltsfoot syrup helps to
calm coughs

The Breathing Process

Air passes into our lungs through the bronchial tubes. Mucus and cilia in the bronchi and lungs help to keep our lungs clear. They do this by sweeping out any unwanted particles. Oxygen is absorbed into the bloodstream in our lungs, and is then carried by the circulatory

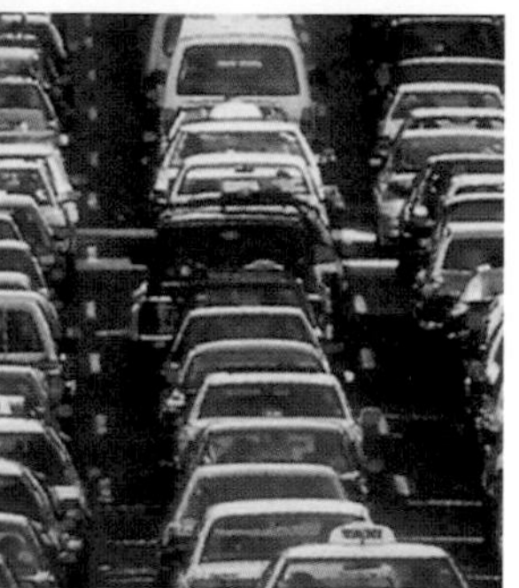

Above The lungs help to filter the air we breathe, allowing fresh oxygen into the bloodstream and protecting us from pollutants. Higher incidences of asthma and other lung diseases can be related to cigarette smoke and traffic fumes.

system into every cell of our body to help release the energy stored in the blood. The waste product of this process is carbon dioxide, which is brought back to our lungs and then exhaled. We breathe in and out about ten to fifteen times a minute, without having to make a conscious effort. This involves enough air to blow up several thousand balloons a day.

Smoking and Pollution

What we breathe becomes a part of us. Cigarette smoke and car fumes are irritants which affect people who suffer from respiratory conditions such as asthma and hayfever. Smoking also contributes to many of the chronic lung conditions, such as lung cancer and emphysema. High levels of pollution in our cities and smoking in the home affect the onset of respiratory diseases in children. There has been an alarming rise in the number of asthmatic children who are dependent on daily doses of steroids in order to breathe.

Prevention of Respiratory Disease

Our lifestyle has become more sedentary, and it is now necessary to make a conscious effort to exercise. Our children, especially, need to be able to run around in the fresh air—something that is becoming more difficult to do with the widespread increase in pollution. Exercise can help to strengthen our lungs. Aerobic exercise forces us to breathe more deeply and fully as the demand for oxygen in the body is increased. Yoga and meditation focus specifically on the way we breathe, helping us to be aware of the expansion and relaxation of the muscles in our chest so that our breathing is less constricted.

The Chinese Medicine Approach

In traditional Chinese medicine, good, strong, healthy lungs are linked with a strong protective *qi*, or energy. Our lungs help us to fight off viruses and infections before they take hold in the body. The traditional Chinese philosophy is that we receive inspiration through the air we breathe. The lung is related to the metal element, the season of autumn (when a lot of us come down with colds), the color white, and the emotion of grief. An old Chinese saying is that catarrh is unshed tears.

Respiratory Ailments

Ailments affecting the respiratory system are very common. Often these complaints are treated with antibiotics. Herbal remedies can sometimes offer a very effective alternative treatment, especially if they are taken at the first signs of illness. In this section, remedies for colds, influenza, sore throats, fevers, sinusitis, tonsillitis, and coughs will be discussed, as well as some for asthma and hayfever.

Colds

Symptoms of a common cold include sneezing, slight chills and fever, scratchy throat, and plenty of catarrh. For most people a cold is merely a discomfort; however, the elderly, babies, and asthmatics need to be careful as a common cold could lead to a more serious chest infection. You can catch a cold when you are under stress or run down and your resistance is low. A cold may be an indication that we need to slow down and rest. A few days off work and some herbal teas can be very effective treatments.

Herbal Treatment There are many herbs that are useful in relieving cold symptoms. An infusion of peppermint, elderflower, and yarrow is helpful (see Herbal Methods chapter pp.20–47). Peppermint has a stimulating, decongestant action; elderflower is drying and anti-catarrhal; and yarrow is a diaphoretic, which means it helps to clear the virus through sweating.

Chinese Herbal Treatment In Chinese medicine, colds are said to be due to an invasion of wind, cold, or heat. If our defenses are low we are more prone to give in to this invasion. If we are tired and exposed to a cold wind, we will end up catching a chill, sneezing, and develop a runny nose. A fever, hot, dry sore throat, and catarrh may follow this. When these symptoms appear, the wind and heat are said to have invaded our body.

The patent remedy *Yin Qiao Jie Du Pien* is famous for getting rid of colds. The two main herbs are *jin yin hua* (honeysuckle) and *lian qiao* (forsythia). These help to clear mild chills and fever, thirst, headache, and cough. It has to be taken with the first signs of a cold, within the first few days of symptoms of sneezing and sore throat, before there is a lot of catarrh. Take one teaspoonful of each herb (make sure you use the Chinese herbs) and put them into a teapot with a cup of boiling water. Let it stand for 10 minutes, then drink. Sweeten with honey if desired. Take three times a day.

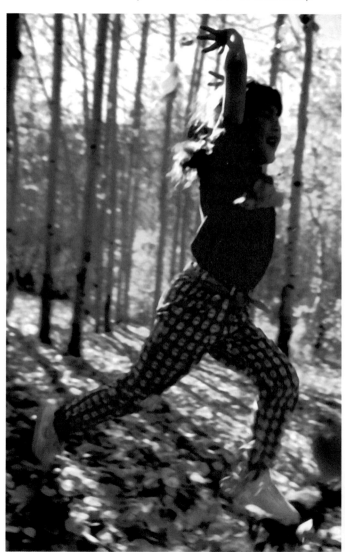

Right Physical exercise helps to strengthen the body, forcing the lungs to breathe deeply and encouraging the circulation. It plays an important role in a healthy childhood.

Fever

Fever or high body temperature is a natural response to infection. It is the body's way of clearing a virus or bacterial infection through perspiration. As viruses and bacteria are broken down by the cells of the immune system, toxins called pyrogens are released. These cause an increase in the body's metabolism and temperature. They are then sweated out through the skin. A normal body temperature is between 96.8–98.6°F (36–37°C). A fever occurs when the temperature rises above 100°F (37.8°C). If the temperature rises above 103°F (38°C), and does not decrease despite efforts to reduce it, or if there are signs of convulsions, fits, or a stiff neck, you should consult a doctor immediately.

Herbal Treatment It is important to drink fluids with a fever to help the body flush out the infection. Try an infusion of camomile or limeflower, which are relaxants as well as diaphoretics. These will help ensure a good sleep, which will help speed recovery. Another delicious tea can be made from one teaspoon of grated ginger and one cinnamon stick infused in one cup of boiling water, with some lemon and honey to taste. This tea encourages sweating and is full of vitamin C, which helps to fight off infections.

Influenza

If a cold and fever continue over several days, and are accompanied by headache and muscular aches and pains, symptoms of flu have developed. A useful herb for these symptoms is boneset, which will quickly relieve aches and pains, as well as help the body to cope with a fever. It will also help to clear any mucus congestion in the upper respiratory tract, as well as constipation. Use an infusion of the dried or fresh herb. Drink one cup of tea every hour, or as often as possible. Combine boneset with elderflower, yarrow, or ginger, depending on your symptoms. Add lemon and honey for flavor, and for additional vitamin C.

Influenza and Depression

If there are signs of depression, which sometimes accompanies influenza, add skullcap to an equal measure of boneset.

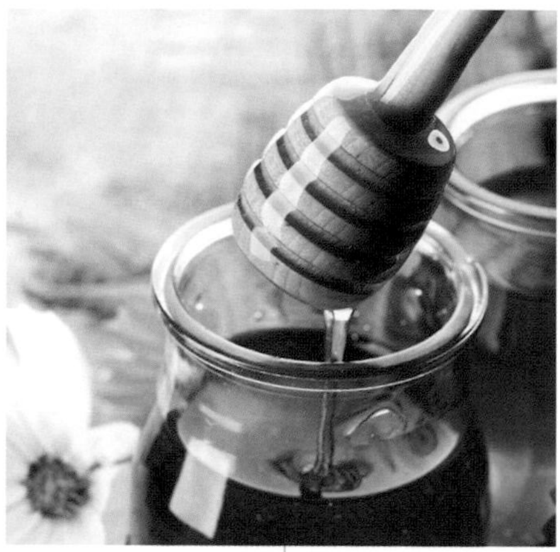

Above Honey is naturally healing and antiseptic. Add it to your herb tea to soothe a sore throat.

Sore Throat

A sore throat may be the first sign of an infection. If it is accompanied by cold symptoms, use the herbs suggested for colds to help clear it. A gargle can also be made using a tea of red sage, thyme, or goldenseal. All these herbs have antiseptic properties and will help fight infections. Gargle with these herbs three to six times a day. Just a word of warning: goldenseal is an excellent herb, but it is very bitter and should be used only in small amounts. It should also be avoided during pregnancy.

The Protective Role of the Tonsils

The tonsils are part of the lymphatic system and have a protective role in defending the body against infection and pollution. They also act as a filter of poisons in the bloodstream and those draining from the nose and sinuses. Inflammation of the tonsils indicates an increased fight to rid the body of toxins and infections. Herbal treatment aims at supporting their work, as well as easing the pain, redness, and swelling of tonsillitis.

Acute Tonsillitis

Acute tonsillitis flares up quickly with a painful and red throat. Most commonly it is a response to a bacterial infection. Use the herbs suggested above for sore throats to ease the discomfort and to soothe the sinus membranes. A gargle of marshmallow tea can soothe a scratchy and burning throat. You should also drink a tea which helps to clear infections: use a mixture of echinacea, calendula, cleavers, and camomile. The echinacea will help to boost the immune system, the calendula and cleavers support the lymphatic tissue in its cleansing work, and the camomile is calming and helps to reduce fevers.

Sinus Infections

Sinusitis is an infection of the sinus cavities, with symptoms of headache pain and a blocked or runny nose.

Herbal Treatment For acute sinusitis, use a combination of echinacea to boost the immune system; goldenseal to help clear the catarrh; and marshmallow leaves to soothe the sinus membranes. Avoid goldenseal if you are pregnant. Try substituting one teaspoonful of elderflower instead. If there is a fever, add yarrow to the infusion.

Steam Inhalation A steam inhalation of aromatic herbs such as eucalyptus and pine needles can help to clear the sinuses. Put three teaspoonfuls of leaves in a basin, and add 4 pints (2 liters) of boiling water. Inhale the steam through the nose for about 10 minutes (see Herbal Methods chapter, pp.20–47). Do not go outside immediately after treatment as the mucus membranes will be very sensitive.

Dietory Factors and Herbal Treatment Take a combination of cleavers and calendula as a tincture or tea for a period of several weeks to help clear the sinuses. In cases of chronic sinusitis, it is necessary to look at the diet. An allergy to dairy products may cause an excessive amount of catarrh to be produced, continually inflaming the mucus membranes. Environmental factors, such as dust and pollution, should also be taken into account.

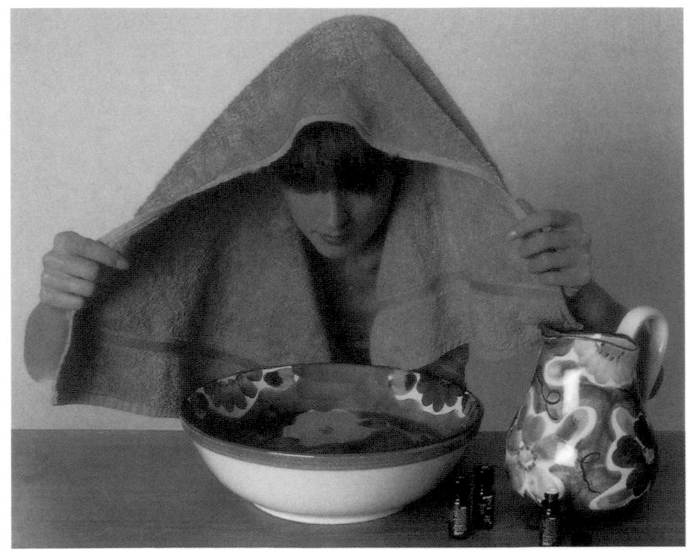

Left A steam inhalation of aromatic herbs, such as pine or eucalyptus, helps to open and clear blocked sinuses.

Coughs

Coughs are the body's attempt to remove obstruction in the throat and chest. Many herbs can be used to clear the throat and chest of irritation, phlegm, and infection, and to build up the immune system. Consult the Herbal Directory (see pp.164–215) and make up a tea from a mixture of herbs to help the particular type of cough.

Dry Coughs

For a dry, irritating cough, it is beneficial to take soothing, moistening herbs such as marshmallow, coltsfoot, and hyssop.

Phlegmy Coughs

When the cough has loosened and is producing more phlegm, try a mixture of expectorant herbs such as hyssop, elecampane, and thyme, which should also help to relax the chest and ease coughing spasms. If there is a lot of clear, runny catarrh use ginger and cinnamon to warm and dry it up. A tea of ginger, honey, and lemon will help relieve a cough and cold with chills.

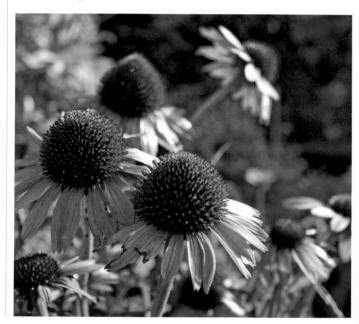

Right Echinacea is popularly believed to act as an immunostimulator, stimulating the body's non-specific immune system and warding off infections.

Chest Infections

If there are signs of a chest infection, such as fever, pain with coughing, and green phlegm, use a combination of echinacea with either elderflower, yarrow, or limeflower. If fever is persistently high or breathing is difficult, seek professional medical help.

Asthma

Over the last two decades there has been a dramatic rise in diagnosed cases of asthma. Many people treat their asthma successfully by using steroid inhalers. Herbal treatment can be used alongside other medication to help reduce the need for these drugs, and to prevent the onset of colds and coughs, which can aggravate asthma attacks. Herbal treatment needs to take place over several months in order to be effective. Any reduction in medication should be done only with professional medical advice.

Dietary Factors Asthma attacks can be triggered by allergic reactions to foods. The most common food allergens are dairy produce, wheat, oranges, eggs, artificial colorings, and preservatives (especially sulfur). Avoid eating one of these foods for several weeks and note if there is any difference in the number of attacks, breathlessness, or vitality.

Environmental Factors The house dustmite is another common cause of asthma, and is prevalent in modern homes which have central heating and carpets. Pets and animals can also trigger wheezing and asthma attacks.

Herbal Treatment There are a number of herbal prescriptions for asthma, and you should seek professional help from an herbalist before using them. For mild cases, the following herbs will be effective, especially if taken over a period of months: echinacea, borage, and licorice will all support the immune system and adrenal glands, which are often low in asthmatics. Combine one of these with coltsfoot, hyssop, elecampane, and thyme. Together these four herbs will help to clear the phlegm and strengthen the lungs. If stress and tension are a factor, add skullcap, vervain, or camomile. These are relaxants, which may help the breathing to become slower and deeper.

Opposite Trees, grasses, and flowers can cause the allergic reactions such as sneezing, runny nose, and red, itchy eyes. Herbal treatment for these symptoms of hayfever can be very effective.

Chinese Herbal Treatment Traditional Chinese herbal medicine has much to offer in the treatment of asthma. There is not enough space here to mention the dried herbs used, but *ma huang* is especially effective for attacks. This herb should only be used under the guidance of an herbalist. The patent remedy *Qing Qi Hua Tan Wan* (Clean Air Tea) is used when there is phlegm that feels stuck in the chest, causing wheeziness. It can help to move the phlegm and open the chest. The formula *Sang Ju Yin* is useful to treat the first symptoms of a cold that goes straight onto the chest.

Hayfever

Hayfever is an allergic reaction to various plant pollens. It is best to start treatment a few months before the hayfever season begins. Taking daily decoctions of echinacea or ginseng can help to build up the immune system and prevent allergic responses. Another interesting treatment is to take a dessertspoonful of honey with the honeycomb with each meal for a month before the season begins. Continue throughout the spring and summer.

Treating Symptoms Once the allergic reactions begin, a combination of elderflower, eyebright, and camomile can be added to the treatment. The elderflower helps to dry the catarrh, the eyebright strengthens the eyes, and the camomile soothes the inflammation.

Chinese Herbal Treatment An excellent Chinese herbal remedy is the patent formula *Bi Yan Pian*. This formula helps to clear the nose, stop sneezing, cool and soothe the eyes, and remove heat caused by the inflammation of the mucus membranes.

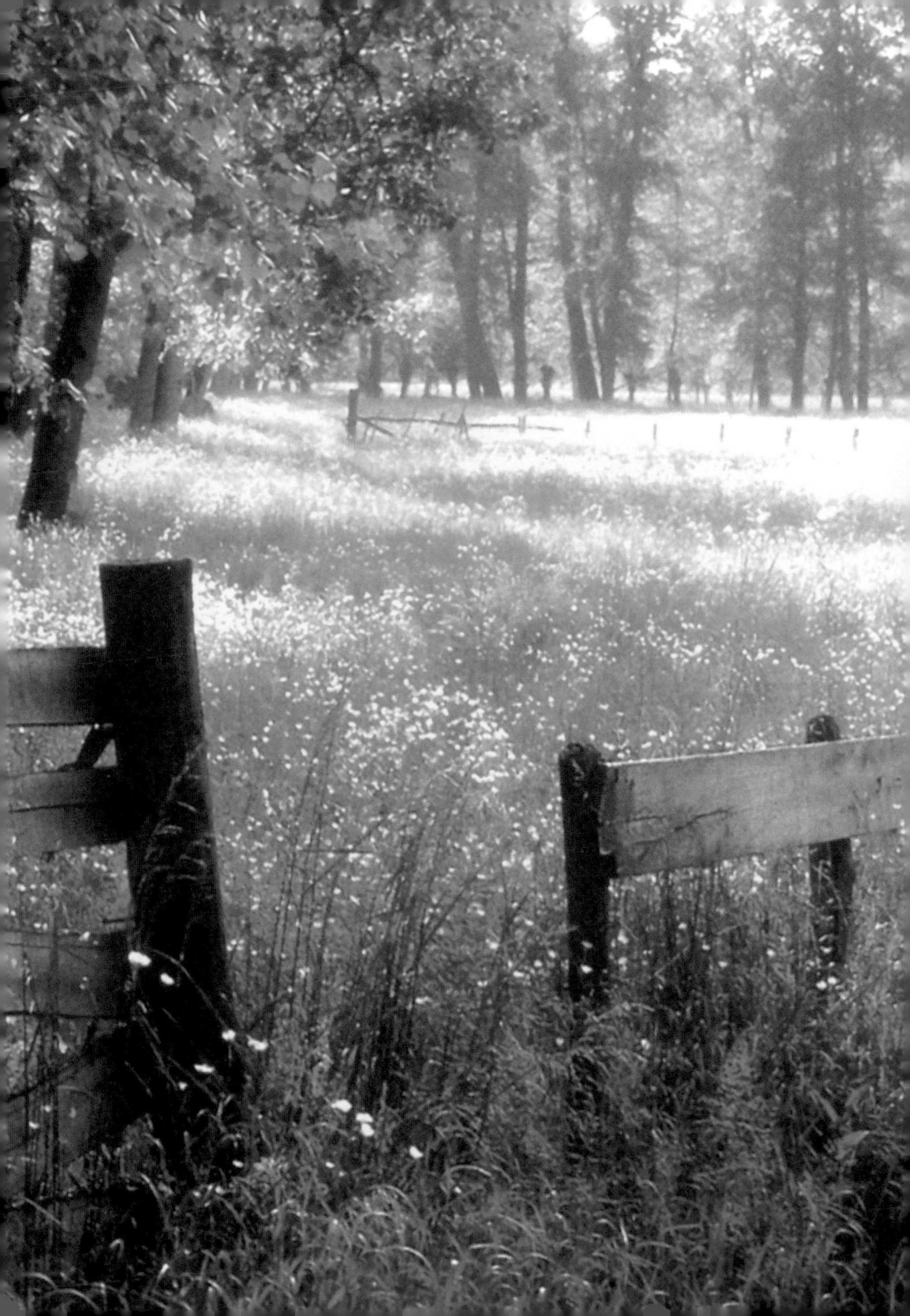

The Eyes and Ears

Sight and hearing, along with the other senses of taste, touch, and smell, help us to perceive and understand the world around us. However, it is all too easy to take these precious abilities for granted. When they are taken from us, due to accident or illness, we can often be left struggling as we learn how to cope.

Many eye and ear problems can be helped by herbal treatment, especially if they are diagnosed early. Herbal treatments are gentle yet they can be highly effective for acute complaints such as conjunctivitis, styes, ear infections, and earache. Chronic eye conditions, glue ear, and tinnitus require long-term treatment, but they also may respond well to herbs.

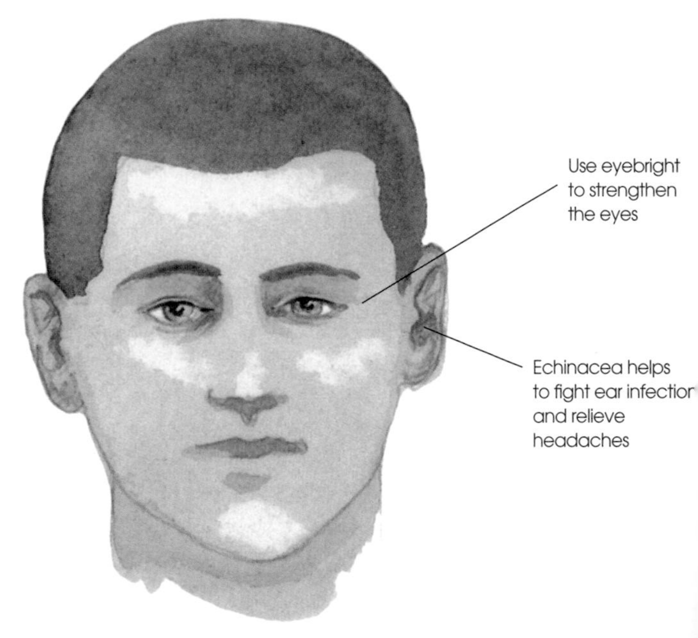
Use eyebright to strengthen the eyes
Echinacea helps to fight ear infectior and relieve headaches

Ailments

Complaints that affect the eyes and ears are extremely common and it is worth trying out the range of herbal treatments detailed here. They can often be highly effective. In this section remedies for all the commonest eye complaints are given: conjunctivitis and blepharitis, styes, chronic eye conditions such as glaucoma and cataracts, and earache, glue ear and tinnitus.

Conjunctivitis and Blepharitis

If you suffer from conjunctivitis the eye becomes irritated because of an infection, an allergy such as hayfever, or pollution. Blepharitis is a more serious condition in which the eyelids become red and inflamed. Take a mixture of echinacea and eyebright as a tea three times a day or as pills to help boost immunity and detoxify the system. If the conjunctivitis is due to allergies, drink a tea of eyebright, camomile, and yarrow three times a day. To ease inflammation, place wet camomile teabags on the closed eyes for 10 minutes.

Herbal Eyewash To relieve symptoms of conjunctivitis or blepharitis bathe the eyes regularly using an eyewash of eyebright tea. Make sure you use a sterilized eyebath and a separate solution and towel for each eye, as these conditions are highly contagious.

Chinese Herbal Treatment The Chinese herb *ju hua* is also said to be very effective in relieving symptoms of dry, red eyes with a sensitivity to light. *Ju hua and* Chrysanthemum tea can be drunk regularly to help the eyes, as well as some headaches.

Styes

Styes are infections at the base of the eyelashes. They are usually an indication of being tired or rundown. They are highly contagious, so it is important to use separate towels when washing. Apply warm compresses (see Herbal Methods chapter, pp.20–47) of eyebright, burdock, or calendula tea frequently throughout the day until the stye bursts or is reabsorbed by the body. Take echinacea, garlic, or goldenseal to help clear the infection.

Chronic Eye Conditions

Chronic eye conditions such as glaucoma, cataracts, and macular degeneration need long-term treatment under professional medical supervision. Herbal treatment, as well as advice on vitamins and minerals from a professional herbalist, can help prevent and slow down deterioration. Antioxidants and bilberry will help to delay macular degeneration and increase visual acuity.

Chinese Herbal Treatment Two well-known traditional Chinese patent formulae that are useful are *Qi Ju Di Huang Wan* and *Ming Mu Di Huang Wan.* They are good for chronic conditions (see Chinese Patent Formulas, pp.43–47). Do not stop any medication prescribed by your doctor without his or her consent; the herbs are to be used as supplements only.

Right Eyebright soothes eye complaints. The parts used include the leaf, the stem, and parts of the flowers. Typical preparations include a warm compress or tea.

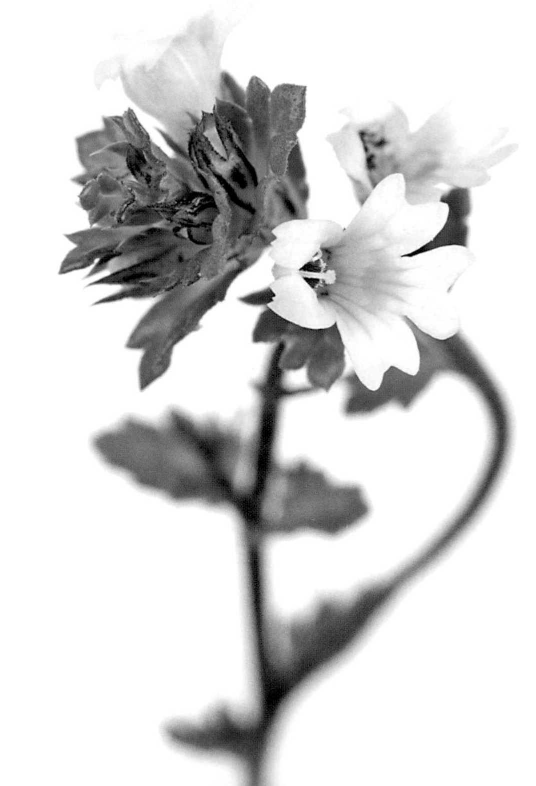

Below Tinnitus and chronic ear infections can result in hearing loss, interfering with the pleasure and necessity of hearing sounds around us. Herbal remedies can be helpful in the treatment of these conditions.

Ear Infections

Infections of the ear often start in the throat and spread through the eustachian tube. Herbal remedies that are anti-microbial and anti-catarrhal, such as goldenseal and echinacea, should be taken as a pill, tea, or tincture. Garlic should be added to food or taken as garlic perles. For external use, first warm the garlic perle in your hands, then place a few drops of garlic oil from it in the ear, provided there is no skin irritation in the ear canal. Keep the oil in with a cotton plug.

Earache

Relieve the pain of an ear infection with a few drops of warm mullein oil or almond oil, or a few drops from a strong infusion of camomile, yarrow, or hyssop tea. If there is much pain, a high fever, or thick discharge from the ear, call your doctor immediately.

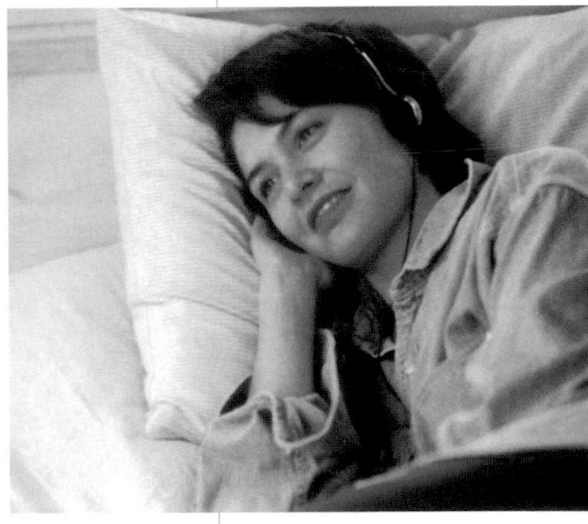

Glue Ear

Chronic ear infections can result in a condition whereby the hearing is diminished by wax and catarrh stuck in the middle ear. Lymphatic tonics, such as cleavers and calendula, need to be used with herbs such as elderflower, goldenseal, and hyssop, which help to clear catarrh. Treatment may need to take place over several months. For children, tinctures are often easier to give. A dairy-free diet may need to be tried for several weeks, since dairy products often cause the body to produce more mucus.

Tinnitus

Tinnitus creates the symptom of noises in the ear. Regular use of goldenseal or black cohosh taken over a period of time may help to relieve these. The traditional Chinese patent remedy *Lui Wei Di Huang Wan* may help, especially with the elderly. A variation called *Er Ming Zuo Ci Wan* may help if the tinnitus is related to high blood pressure. Ginkgo will help to decrease tinnitus for most people, but it needs to be taken for up to three months for results to be experienced.

The Digestive System

Our health and vitality depend on eating a well-balanced diet and the functioning of an efficient digestive system. Absorption of essential nutrients supplies the body with the necessary building blocks to keep it fit and strong.

Interaction with the Body

A good digestive system is a key factor in maintaining health and well-being. If the digestive system is weak or upset, we can feel tired, irritable, and be unable to concentrate and sleep. If bowel elimination is upset, essential food nutrients can be lost, for example in cases of duodenal ulcers and chronic diarrhea. Constipation can give rise to many other complaints, such as low immunity and headaches, due to toxins not being evacuated from the body.

The Chinese Medicine Approach

In traditional Chinese medicine digestion plays an important role in the good health of the body. The stomach and spleen are the main organs related to the digestive system.They have a vital part in the production of *qi*, or energy. The protective *qi*, or *wei qi*, which is the basis for our immune system, is dependent on strong digestion. It is interesting that recent scientific investigations have found a strong correlation between a good immune system and a healthy digestive system.

Prevention of Digestive Disorders

Many disorders of the digestive system can be helped by a careful diet and good eating habits. Meals should be eaten regularly, with breakfast being as important as other meals. Meal times should be relaxed. Time should be allowed to chew food properly, and to allow it to be digested. The diet should include fresh fruit, vegetables, and natural cereals to provide nutrients and roughage. Sugar, starches, and refined flour should be kept to a minimum, and artificial additives should be avoided. Coffee, tea, alcohol, and smoking should also be restricted as they upset the digestive system.

How the Digestive System Works

Food is broken down into a few simple forms which the body is able to utilize to provide the raw materials and energy for cellular activity.

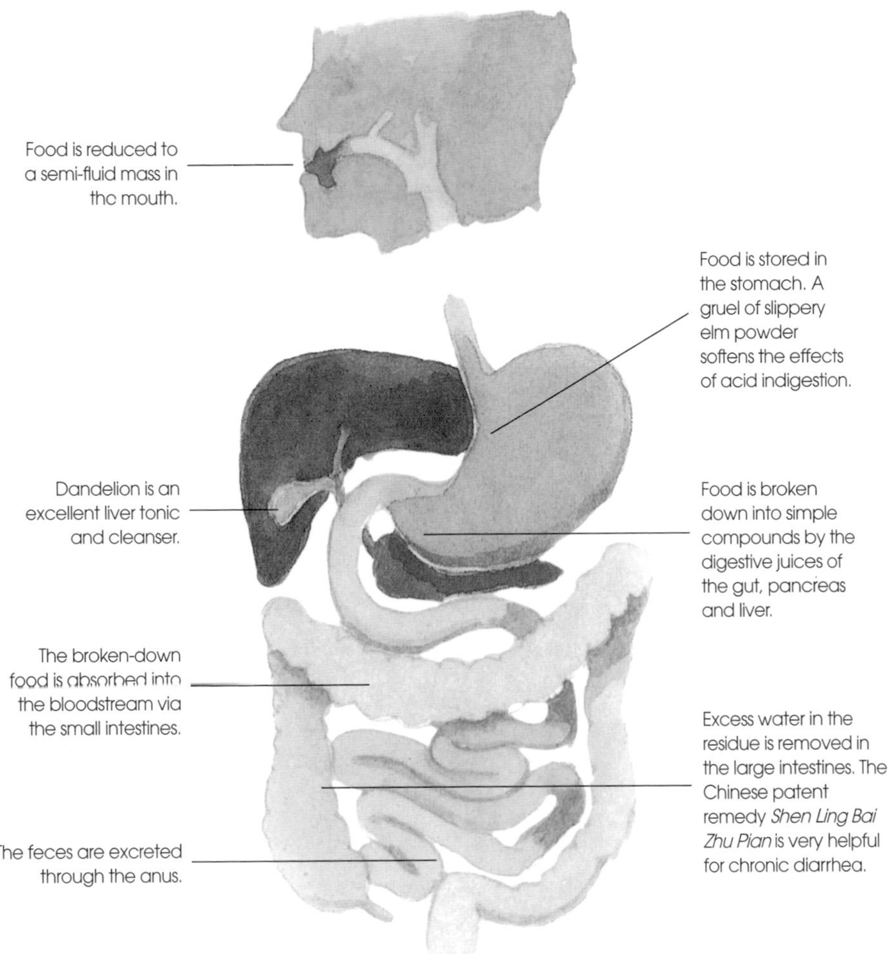

Food is reduced to a semi-fluid mass in the mouth.
Food is stored in the stomach. A gruel of slippery elm powder softens the effects of acid indigestion.
Dandelion is an excellent liver tonic and cleanser.
Food is broken down into simple compounds by the digestive juices of the gut, pancreas and liver.
The broken-down food is absorbed into the bloodstream via the small intestines.
Excess water in the residue is removed in the large intestines. The Chinese patent remedy *Shen Ling Bai Zhu Pian* is very helpful for chronic diarrhea.
The feces are excreted through the anus.

The digestive system begins in the mouth, where food is chewed and mixed with enzymes in the saliva to break it down. It passes through the esophagus to the stomach. Here, food is partly digested through the action of more enzymes, and strong acid secretions, which kill any harmful bacteria. In the small intestine or duodenum, the food is mixed with enzyme-rich secretions from the pancreas and gut wall, and with bile from the liver. Essential nutrients are absorbed into the bloodstream and taken to the liver, where they are processed. In the large intestine or colon, the fluids are absorbed into the bloodstream, leaving the residue, or fecal matter, to be expelled when convenient.

The Effect of Stress and Tension

The digestive system is richly supplied with nerves, making it prone to the effects of stress and nervous tension. The autonomic nervous system regulates the blood supply to and from the digestive system, as well as the production of the digestive juices. The digestive system is susceptible to our thoughts and emotions, which is why we use the phrase "gut reaction."

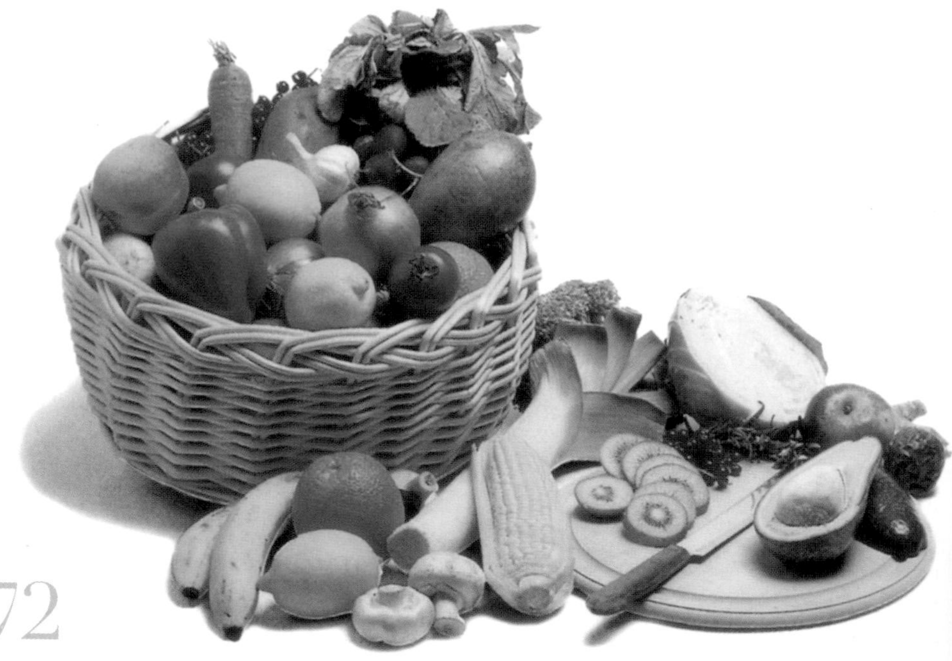

Below A healthy diet of fresh foods including fruits and vegetables will provide nutrients and roughage. Good eating habits are important to help maintain a strong digestive system.

Digestive Ailments

In this section, ailments relating to the whole digestive system, such as constipation, diarrhea, nausea and vomiting, and gastric pain are discussed. The digestive system is then divided into its parts, so that ailments relating more specifically to the mouth, stomach, small intestines, and large intestines are reviewed. Herbal treatments, along with some dietary advice, are suggested for each ailment discussed.

Constipation

Eating too much refined food and not enough fruits, vegetables, and wholegrains, which contain roughage, is a major cause of constipation. Lack of exercise, stress, and food allergies can also cause it. In chronic constipation, the muscles of the bowel need to be stimulated to push the stools out. Long-term use of laxatives can block this natural movement (peristalsis). With aging, the bowel can become weak and sluggish, needing more roughage and moisture to help the contents move through smoothly.

Herbal Treatment Gentle remedies such as linseed and psyllium seeds can help to provide bulk and roughage. Soak one or two teaspoonfuls of these seeds in 8 fl oz (200 ml) of hot water for two hours. Add lemon and honey for flavor, and drink before bedtime. If necessary, another drink can be taken first thing in the morning as well. Linseed can also be added to a bowl of wholegrain cereal for breakfast. A decoction of more stimulating laxative herbs can be taken for up to two weeks. Use a combination of licorice, dandelion root, yellow dockroot, burdock, and ginger. If stress and tension are involved, add camomile or crampbark. If constipation persists or is painful, seek professional medical advice.

Diarrhea

Acute diarrhea is the body's way of eliminating poisons or infections. It can occur with food poisoning or stomach bugs. For mild diarrhea, drink a tea of meadowsweet to soothe and calm the gut. If it is related to an infection, drink teas of camomile, thyme, ginger, or fennel, either on their own or in combination to help fight the infection and relieve ache and discomfort. Sometimes bouts of diarrhea can be due to nervous tension. In this case, drink teas of camomile or lemon balm combined with meadowsweet to help relax the gut. If diarrhea persists, or if there is blood or mucus in the stools, seek professional medical advice.

A Chinese Remedy The traditional Chinese patent remedy *Shen Ling Bai Zhu Pian* is excellent for chronic diarrhea due to weakness in the digestive system. It helps to tone digestion, and relieve symptoms of belching, bloating, indigestion, and abdominal fullness, as well as loose stools. It can be used with children, and is especially helpful to those who are fussy eaters, or who have allergic reactions to food. It can be used for prolonged periods.

Nausea and Vomiting

Nausea and vomiting can be symptoms of food poisoning, stomach infections, morning sickness, migraine, or nervousness. To help settle the stomach, sip teas of ginger root, peppermint, or camomile. As they all have their own flavor, choose one that suits your individual taste; add honey if preferred. If there is an infection, add tinctures of echinacea or goldenseal to teas of lavender, thyme, or lemon balm.

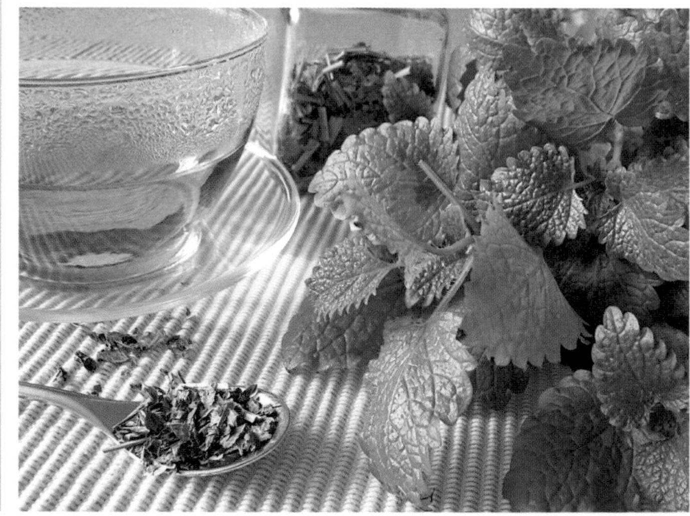

Right Teas and tinctures can be made from a combination of herbs, in this case lemon balm, which is a gentle but effective way to ease the discomfort of digestive complaints.

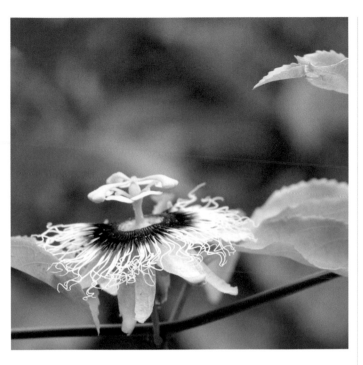

Left Passionflower is an anti-spasmodic herb and has been used for treating digestive discomfort, seizures, hysteria, uterine pains, and aches and pains of all kinds. It is also a well-known tonic for the nervous system, a natural sedative and tranquilizer.

If stress is likely to be a factor, drink teas of camomile, lemon balm, or passionflower to help relax. If vomiting is severe or persistent, call the doctor immediately.

Digestive Pains

Pain in the digestive system can be symptomatic of different problems. Any strong or persistent pains should be investigated by a doctor. Colic and griping pains are usually due to muscle spasms in the gut as it attempts to push its contents through the system. Carminative herbs, such as peppermint, ginger, fennel, lemon balm, and camomile, which are specific for relieving gas and wind, can be taken as a tea or tincture in warm water after meals. Add warming spices, such as cinnamon, ginger, and cardamom to foods to ease the digestion. Massage the abdomen in a clockwise direction with a few drops of warming oils of cinnamon, ginger, cloves, or peppermint diluted in a base oil.

The Mouth

The digestive system begins in the mouth. Problems with the teeth and gums can make the chewing of food difficult. Treatments for toothache, gingivitis, abscesses, and mouth ulcers are suggested below, enabling the whole digestive process to be more efficient. Dental hygiene is an important part of preventative care.

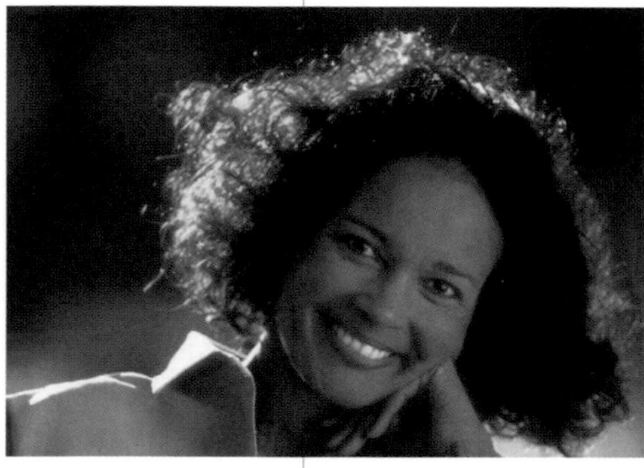

Above A bright smile with healthy gums and teeth is a vital part of our expression. Good dental hygiene reduces the risk of toothache and gum infections.

Toothache

When problems arise, teeth must be treated by a dentist. An herbal first-aid remedy for toothache is to chew some cloves, which contain a pain-relieving oil called eugenol. Alternatively, soak a piece of absorbent cotton (cotton wool) in clove oil and place it next to the tooth. Peppermint oil can also be used, but is not as effective.

Gingivitis

Gingivitis is an infection of the superficial tissue of the gum. It can cause the gums to appear red and swollen and to bleed easily. Much gum disease can be reduced through good oral hygiene and by avoiding sugars and refined, processed foods. Take garlic or echinacea to help fight infections. Rinse the mouth with a teaspoon of a mixture of echinacea and myrrh tinctures in a small amount of water. This does not have a pleasant taste, but is very effective.

Abscesses

A tooth abscess is a very painful condition that must be examined and assessed by the dentist. Antibiotics are the conventional form of treatment, and are usually quite effective. An herbal remedy can be made from a decoction of echinacea, cleavers, and pokeroot, which will help to fight the infection and cleanse the lymphatic system. Garlic perles and high doses of vitamin C are also beneficial.

Mouth Ulcers

Mouth ulcers can indicate that the body is run-down or under stress.

Recovery from colds and flu, or the use of antibiotics and stress can cause an outbreak of mouth ulcers. The whole body should be treated with strengthening and calming teas of ginseng, lemon balm, vervain, and licorice. Coffee, tea, and cigarette smoking should be avoided. Treat the ulcers with a mouthwash of red sage and myrrh. In North America a commercially produced licorice extract called "deglycyrrhizinated licorice," or "DGL," is also used in the treatment of ulcers and hyperacidity.

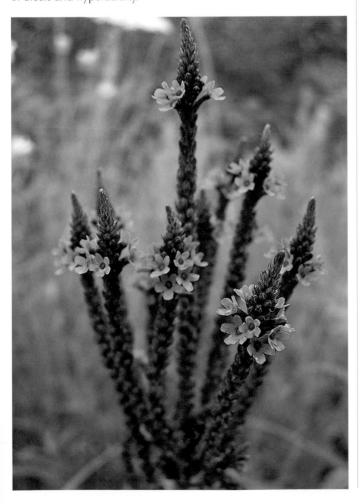

Left Vervain, from the Verbena plant, is an astringent, diaphoretic and antispasmodic. It is said to be useful for treating fevers, ulcers, and ophthalmia.

The Stomach

The main function of the stomach is to digest food using digestive enzymes and hydrochloric acid. Stomach acid helps to break down food and sterilize it so that harmful bacteria are not passed on.

Indigestion

Symptoms of indigestion can vary from pain and heartburn to discomfort and flatulence. They are often triggered by stress and excitement, irregular meals, and over-eating. Being allergic to certain foods will also bring on the symptoms of indigestion. Foods that are rich, fatty, or spicy should be avoided as well as coffee, tea, cigarettes, and alcohol. A change in diet and lifestyle may be required to bring about a long-term cure.

Herbal Treatment With the first sign of discomfort, take slippery elm powder or tablets to soothe the inflamed stomach lining. Drink teas made from a mixture of meadowsweet, marshmallow, and licorice, which will help to reduce stomach acid and heal inflammation. After meals, drink teas of camomile, rosemary, peppermint, and fennel to help settle the stomach and aid digestion. If stress and tension are likely to be a factor, drink teas of camomile, lemon balm, and vervain to aid relaxation.

Gastritis

Gastritis is an irritation of the stomach lining, which can be caused by an infection or a reaction to food. It can start with an acute case of food poisoning or a stomach bug, and last for a while afterward. Gastritis is treated through diet and herbs. Drinks such as coffee, tea, and alcohol, and rich, spicy, and greasy foods should be avoided. With acute inflammation do not eat foods high in fiber or acid, such as bran, nuts, seeds, tomatoes, vinegar, and pickles. Do not smoke, as this increases the production of stomach acid.

Herbal Treatment A decoction of the following herbs will help to soothe and heal the stomach lining. Use a mixture of one part marshmallow root and meadowsweet to one half-part goldenseal. The goldenseal has a powerful healing quality for the membranes of the stomach lining, but as it also stimulates the muscles of the uterus, it should be avoided during pregnancy. If stress and tension are aggravating the gastritis, add valerian to the decoction. Drink this tea after each meal until the condition clears.

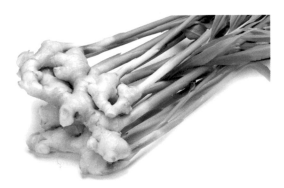

Above Ginger, or ginger root, helps protect and heal the gut. Ginger also treats a broader range of inflammatory problems. It can also relieve nausea and destroy a number of viruses.

Gastric Ulcer

A gastric ulcer occurs when the mucus membranes of the stomach lining break down and the digestive juices start to irritate the stomach wall. Herbal treatment is similar to gastritis. Take a decoction of marshmallow root, meadowsweet, and goldenseal. The marshmallow root soothes and heals the stomach membranes. The meadowsweet helps to settle the stomach and slow the production of acid. The goldenseal is beneficial to the mucus membranes, but should be avoided in pregnancy. Take slippery elm as a powder or tablet morning and night to help protect the stomach from acid.

Dietary Factors If a gastric ulcer forms, it is an indication that changes in the diet and lifestyle are needed if the ulcer is to clear permanently. The diet should be low in fiber and protein while the ulcer pain is acute. Eat small, well-cooked meals of easily digestible foods frequently. Avoid alcohol, tea, coffee, and tobacco as well as acidic, spicy, or greasy foods. As the ulcer heals, eat a well-balanced diet, reintroducing fiber and proteins. It is best to seek professional advice for this condition.

Chinese Herbal Treatment *Bu Zhong Yi Qi Wan* is a Chinese patent remedy that helps to strengthen the digestive system. It should not be used with acute conditions, but with more chronic complaints of abdominal bloating, pain, flatulence, and erratic stools. It contains herbs which strengthen the digestion such as astralagus (*huang qi*), licorice (*gan cao*), and ginger root (*sheng jiang*). It also contains herbs that help move the digestive *qi*, or energy, so that feelings of fullness and abdominal bloating are eased.

The Intestines

The small intestine makes up the longest part of the digestive system—its length can be up to 20 feet (60 meters). Its main function is to absorb nutrients from the food into the bloodstream. The large intestine absorbs water and minerals. Bacteria in the gut (gut flora) help to make vitamins and to clear toxic bacteria.

Duodenal Ulcers

The duodenum is the first part of the small intestines. It starts below the pyloric sphincter, which is the valve that separates the stomach and small intestines. If it does not function properly, acid from the stomach leaks into the alkaline environment of the small intestines and can cause an ulcer.

Herbal Treatment Make a decoction of marshmallow and licorice root with meadowsweet and goldenseal to help heal and soothe the damaged lining. Always refer to the contraindications in the Herbal Directory (pp.164–215) before using goldenseal, licorice, or any other herb. Drink this before meals. Slippery elm powder taken as a gruel will help to coat the gut lining and protect it from acidity and irritation. Take this first thing in the morning and last thing at night. Eat little and often, and avoid spicy, fatty, or greasy foods, vinegar, coffee, tea, alcohol, and tobacco. It is best to seek professional advice for treatment for this condition.

Stress and Tension

To relieve feelings of stress and tension that often accompany ulcers, drink relaxing teas of camomile, lemon balm, vervain, and skullcap, which will help to strengthen the nervous system and ease tension. Take an herbal bath with oils or strong infusions of lavender, camomile, and lemon balm.

Irritable Bowel Syndrome (IBS)

The workings of the bowel are susceptible to our emotions. Stress and tension, along with poor eating habits and food intolerances, can aggravate any inflammation and irritation in the lining of the bowel. Symptoms of IBS include alternating diarrhea and constipation, flatulence, and griping pains. This can vary from discomfort to severe pain with diarrhea. Eliminating any suspected food allergies can do a lot to relieve symptoms. The most common ones include tea, coffee, milk, eggs, wheat, or gluten. Any severe pain, or persistent diarrhea or constipation, needs medical attention.

Herbal Treatment Drink a tea made from a combination of wild yam, camomile, peppermint, marshmallow, and goldenseal. The wild yam will help to relieve spasms; the camomile and peppermint will encourage good digestion; the marshmallow will soothe the inflammation; and the goldenseal helps to heal the membranes. Only use goldenseal in small doses, and do not use it at all if you are pregnant. Drink the tea three times a day over a period of time. Another helpful tip might to substitute coffee and tea with simple herbal teas of camomile, lemon balm, and fennel. These will help you to relax and ease tension.

Herbal Treatment The Chinese patent formula *Xiao Yao Wan* (Free and Easy Wanderer) is helpful in cases of IBS, especially if it is worse during times of stress and accompanies PMS. It helps to relax the *qi*, or energy, and encourages digestion. It is useful with symptoms of abdominal bloating, fullness, and poor appetite, and those symptoms which are related to food allergies.

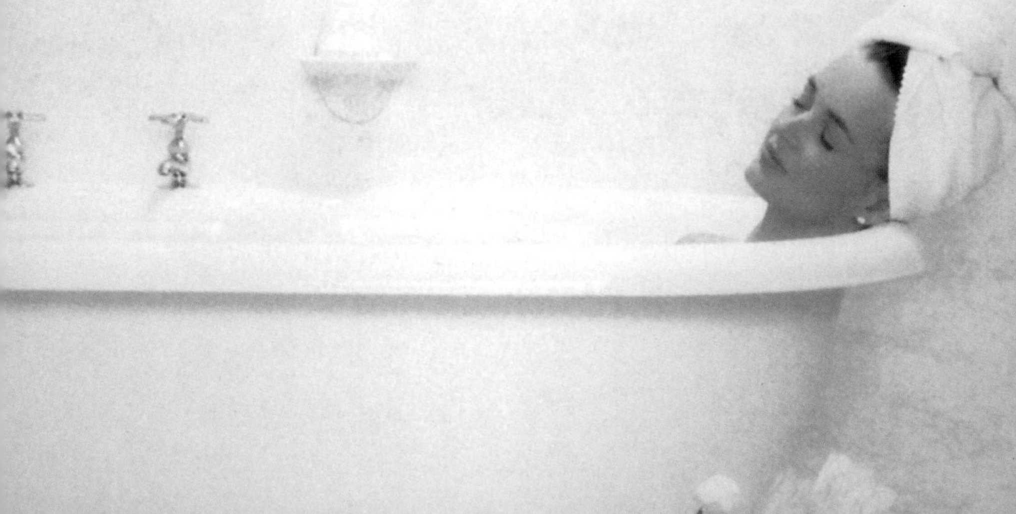

Below An herbal bath with strong infusions of lavender, camomile, and lemon balm will help to relieve stress that may aggravate digestive complaints. Take a relaxing bath to soothe away cares and tension.

Hemorrhoids

Hemorrhoids, or piles, is a painful condition related to the blood vessels of the rectum and anus. The most common cause is chronic constipation, and if this can be avoided, the piles will be relieved. A simple infusion of the herb pilewort may tone the vessels and ease their inflammation. The astringent qualities of witch hazel, which can be made into a suppository (see Herbal Methods chapter, pp.20–47), will also help to shrink and relieve pain.

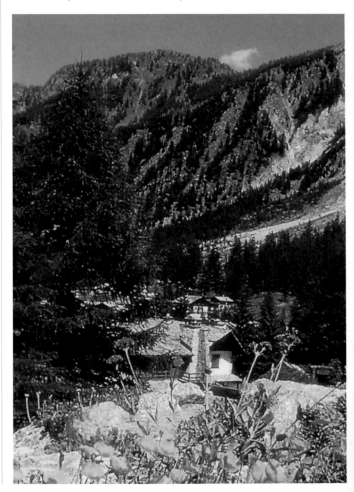

Below Herbal folklore suggests a "spring tonic" to cleanse and revitalize the body after a winter lacking in physical exercise and fresh foods.

The Liver and Gall Bladder

The liver is the largest organ inside the body, and plays a vital role in the digestive process. It is involved in the processing of carbohydrates and is the most important organ in maintaining blood sugar levels. It helps to break down proteins and fats. It stores vitamins A, D, K, and B12. The fat-soluble vitamins depend on bile, which is produced in the liver, for their absorption.

The liver also helps to regulate hormones. It detoxifies drugs and other chemicals; helping to keep the body clear and well-functioning. The liver produces and secretes bile, which is stored in the gallbladder. Bile helps to break down and absorb fats, as well as activate the pancreas.

Herbal Treatment for the Liver

Spring tonics are part of folk remedy tradition, and are used to cleanse and support the liver after a winter of poor food. They are still relevant for the stresses of modern life. Pollution, food additives, greasy fast foods, and drug and alcohol abuse all put strain on the liver. A useful liver tonic can be made from dandelion, meadowsweet, and goldenseal. The roots and leaves of dandelion make a good tonic and cleanser for the liver and the kidneys; meadowsweet will support the stomach; and goldenseal (use in small doses and avoid if pregnant) helps to tone and stimulate the digestive system. Milk thistle is another excellent herb which supports and helps to cleanse the liver. Drink 4 pints (2 liters) of water a day to flush the system, and avoid eating any fried, roasted, or fatty foods.

Below Liver and gallbladder problems are treated with meadowsweet tea; it is said to promote the flow of bile.

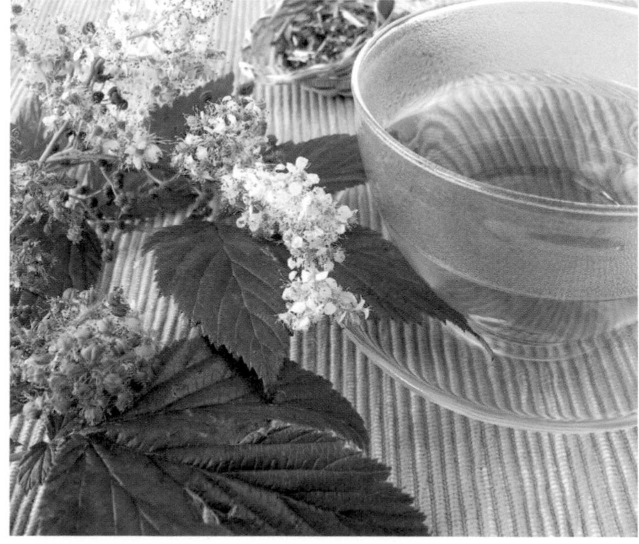

The Urinary System

The urinary system has the important task of regulating the amount of water in the body and producing urine to carry away waste products. Its functioning is vital to keeping the body healthy and fit by preventing dehydration and a buildup of toxic material.

The kidneys and bladder are the two main organs of the urinary system. The kidneys work to regulate water in the body, filter and cleanse the blood, and restore body fluids to a pure and useful state. Waste is passed out through the urine, which leaves the kidneys via the ureters to the bladder, where it is stored. It is then discharged out of the body through the urethra. In this section herbal treatment for discomforts such as cystitis and urethritis will be discussed, as well as other related problems, such as water retention and incontinence. More serious conditions, such as prostate and kidney problems, may require advice from a professional herbalist, but some supportive herbal treatments are suggested.

The Kidneys

The renal artery brings circulating blood to the kidneys for filtering. This is a complex process, which involves the absorption of essential nutrients, cleansing of wastes, and reabsorption of nutrients into the body. The kidneys also help maintain the acid-alkaline balance of the blood, and regulate the salt balance within the body. The adrenal glands, which produce adrenaline, are situated on top of the kidneys. They can affect the kidneys' secretion of sodium into the blood, and the production of the hormone renin.

The Chinese Medicine Approach

In traditional Chinese medicine there is a strong link between the kidney and the bladder. They are related to our energy reserves, which are frequently depleted in our society, where there is a strong emphasis on achievement and hard work. The season associated with the water element, which is related to the kidney and bladder, is winter. This is the time for resting and replenishing energy so that there will be a strong start to new growth in the spring. Weak kidney and bladder *qi*, or energy, can be related to many complaints of low-back ache and fatigue, as well as the ailments listed here.

How the Urinary System Works

Nitrogenous wastes (mainly as the simple compound urea) and acids are removed from the blood by the kidneys.

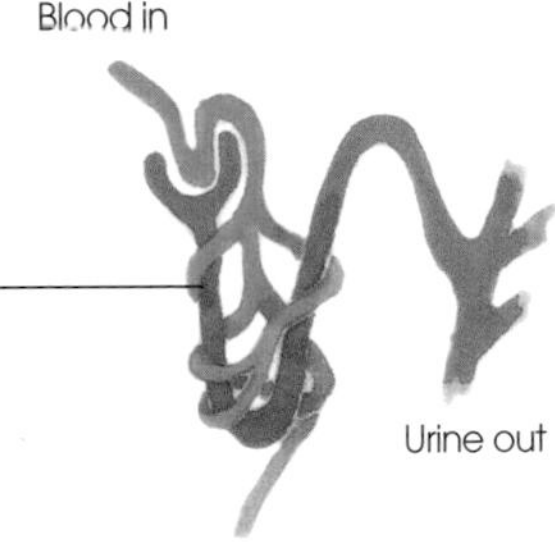

Blood in
Tubules
The fluid part of the blood (free of cells and protein) is filtered under pressure into long tubules in the kidney. The tubules are selectively permeable, and most of the fluid and any essential compounds are reabsorbed back into the blood. For kidney infections , drink an herbal tea of echinacea, celery seed, couchgrass, and yarrow.
Urine
A small fraction of the fluid containing waste matter remains in the tubules and forms the urine.
Urine out
Blood out

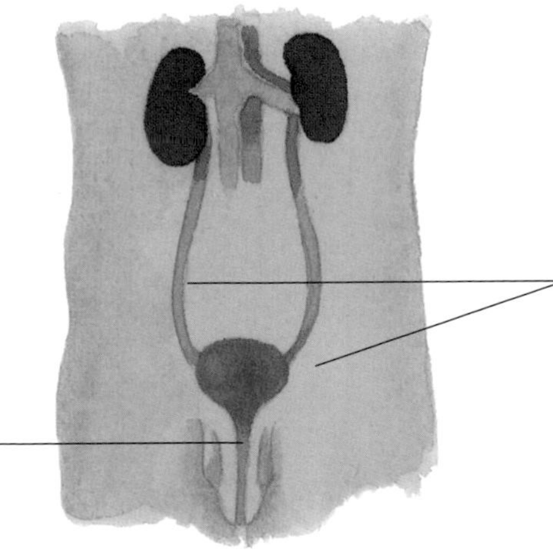

The ureters
Urine passes down the ureters. Barley water helps to alkalize the urine and ease the burning pains of cystitis and urethritis.
The Bladder
From the ureters the urine passes into the bladder and is excreted at intervals. Drink a tea of marshmallow, couchgrass, and yarrow to soothe bladder inflammation.

Urinary Ailments

Healthy functioning of any part of the body relies on the kidneys' ability to eliminate waste products and toxins. Our food and diet tend to contain many chemicals and artificial products, which puts a strain on kidney function. It is important to drink plenty of liquids to help the kidneys flush through toxins and prevent illness. Avoid drinking excessive amounts of alcohol, coffee, and tea to make their job easier. To prevent strain on the bladder, try to pass water when the urge is felt rather than holding out for long periods.

Cystitis and Urethritis

Infection of the bladder or urethra can be a chronic or acute condition. Symptoms include a burning pain on passing urine, often accompanied by pain in the groin during or just after urination. A desire to pass water although the bladder is empty is another common symptom. Drink plenty of water to help clear the infection. Cranberry juice or extract will also help by preventing the bacteria's ability to adhere to the wall of the bladder. Take a tea of marshmallow, couchgrass, and yarrow to soothe the inflammation. If it is at the early stage, which is the best time to treat cystitis, an infusion of yarrow tea drunk three times a day may solve the problem. You can add camomile to help you relax if feelings of anxiety and tension are present. If the burning is very strong, cornsilk may be added. If pain is severe, or there is a fever, seek professional medical help.

Soothing Drink To help alkalize the urine and ease some of the burning, drink barley water throughout the day. Use 4 oz (100 g) of washed barley with 1 pint (600 ml) water. Simmer in a nonaluminum pot with a lid until the barley is soft. Strain and keep the liquid. Add a small amount of honey and lemon, and drink this mixture warm.

Prevention Some women are prone to urinary-tract infection. Any disturbance within the body may start an attack of cystitis or urethritis. Stress, overwork, and antibiotics may lower resistance to infection. In this case it is important to drink at least 2 pints (1 liter) of water daily and urinate frequently. Avoid coffee, sugar, and acidic foods such as tomatoes and citrus fruits. In some individuals, caffeine will prevent the bladder from completely emptying. Deodorant douches and bathing in soapy water may cause irritation, and should be avoided.

Chinese Herbal Treatment There are many useful Chinese herbal remedies for cystitis and urethritis. The remedies vary, depending on whether the symptoms include blood in the urine, cloudy urine, acute pain, or chronic discomfort. *Bu Zhong Yi Qi Wan* is a patent remedy useful in cases of the more chronic type. Symptoms include difficult urination that comes in a weak stream, slight abdominal distension, and general tiredness. This remedy is a general tonic that helps to raise the *qi*, or energy, allowing the infection to clear from the body.

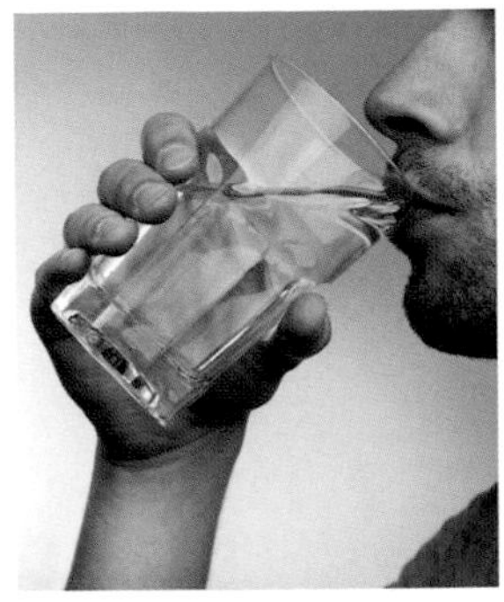

Above Drink plenty of water each day to help support the kidneys' function of clearing the toxins out of the body.

Prostatitis

An infection of the prostate gland is generally not as localized as cystitis, and may need a more overall approach. Echinacea is a good herbal antibiotic, and should be combined with couchgrass, celery seed, and horsetail. Add saw palmetto as a tonic for the male hormone and gland; it helps to shrink the prostate gland. Take as a decoction or tincture three times a day (see Herbal Methods chapter, pp.20–47). For a swollen prostate gland, take a zinc supplement, or eat a handful of pumpkin seeds daily. A teaspoonful of safflower oil or cold-pressed linseed oil daily will help supply essential fatty acids. Drink a decoction of false unicorn root, dandelion, saw palmetto, couchgrass, and prickly ash three times a day. Take plenty of exercise. Any swelling or discomfort of the prostate should be investigated by a doctor.

Water Retention

Water retention can be a symptom of many different problems, from circulation and kidney complaints to hormonal imbalance. It is important to find the cause of the problem, and this may involve medical tests. To treat cases of mild water retention, drink any herbal teas which have diuretic properties, the best ones being dandelion leaf and yarrow (see Herbal Directory, p.206) for more information on the diuretic powers of dandelion.) If there is no improvement in ten days, seek medical attention. If the water retention is part of premenstrual symptoms, add *vitex* to help balance the hormones.

Incontinence

Incontinence has both physical and psychological causes. If there is no major physical defect, herbal treatment may be helpful. It is worth a try in cases where incontinence is due to a loss of tone of the sphincter muscle, or to general muscle or nervous debility. Make a decoction of two parts horsetail and one part agrimony, and drink this three times a day (see Herbal Methods chapter, pp.20–47).

Bedwetting

A child over the age of six who still wets the bed regularly may need medical investigation to see if there is an underlying physical problem. Bedwetting can also be due to stress, anxiety, and food allergies. Avoid giving drinks before bed, take the child to the toilet in the night, and try to encourage dry nights with small rewards. A tea made from St. John's wort, horsetail, and cornsilk sweetened with honey, will help to soothe any irritation in the bladder. Add camomile, skullcap, or lemon balm if the child is stressed or worried.

Chinese Herbal Treatment The Chinese herbal repertory consists mainly of plants; however, it also uses some animal parts, and even stones and minerals. For example, the Chinese herb chicken livers *(ji nei jin)* is a useful remedy for bedwetting in children. It is very effective and easy to give. The chicken livers are available as a powder, which can be mixed into fruit juice or water. Use a teaspoonful of powder daily for several weeks. The remedy can also help with incontinence in adults, and to dissolve urinary stones—but professional advice is needed for both problems.

Kidney Stones

The formation of stones, or mineral deposits, in the kidney responds well to herbal treatment. A low-acid diet is recommended to help stop the stones forming; this means totally avoiding foods high in oxalic acid, such as rhubarb and spinach. Drink up to 6 pints (3 liters) of water a day, preferably one with a low mineral content, to help flush out the system. Take a combination of herbs as a tea or tincture to help dissolve and wash out the stones or gravel. A mixture of couchgrass, dandelion leaves, cleavers, marshmallow, and stone root will help this condition. Extra vitamin B6 and magnesium will prevent new stones forming.

Kidney Infections

Kidney infections are a serious and painful condition, and need professional medical advice. The herbal treatment suggested here can be used to support medical treatment. Drink plenty of liquids, avoiding coffee, tea, and alcohol. Instead, drink camomile and limeblossom tea to help relax and ease pain. Take a mixture of echinacea, celery seed, couchgrass, and yarrow to help fight the infection. Drink 1 pint (600 ml) of tea a day.

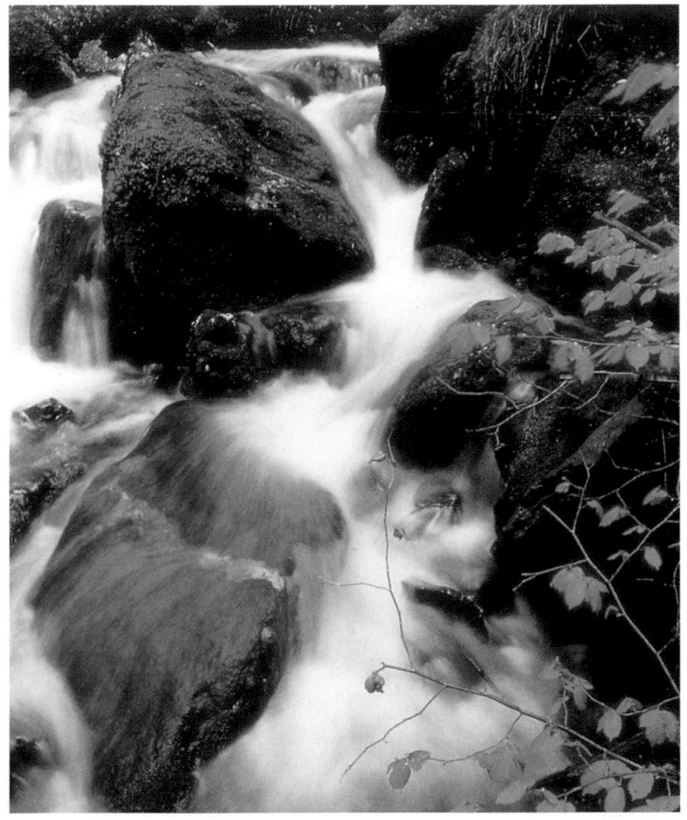

Left A large part of our body is water. Drinking 2 pints (1 liter) of water daily will help to maintain a well-functioning urinary system.

The Reproductive System

The reproductive system is one of nature's most miraculous "inventions," yet it can also cause anguish, pain, and discomfort if there are problems. Primarily the female reproductive system is discussed here, along with some suggestions for herbs to help male impotence and low sperm count.

The primary female reproductive organs are the ovaries, which secrete the hormones progesterone and estrogen and produce the ova, or eggs. Hormones secreted by the pituitary gland interact with those released by the ovaries to create the menstrual cycle. Ovulation occurs about fourteen days into the menstrual cycle. If fertilization occurs, pregnancy begins. If the egg is not fertilized, it is shed with the lining of the uterus at the end of the twenty-eight-day cycle.

Changes in the Menstrual Cycle

From the onset of the menses through to menopause the menstrual cycle varies with each woman. Hormonal changes due to pregnancy and birth, aging, and life events all affect the menstrual cycle. For some women this is not a problem, yet others may need some support for the discomforts brought on by these hormonal changes. Herbal treatment has been used by women for many centuries to help the body to cope with these changes.

The Native American Approach

In Native American tradition, there is a strong relationship with the earth as the mother who looks after us, providing food and a home. Traditionally herbs were seen as part of the earth's gifts. Herb gathering was always done with prayers of thanks, and some of the plant was left to regrow. We should remember this, as some herbs are now scarce due to environmental destruction and over-picking.

How the female reproductive system works

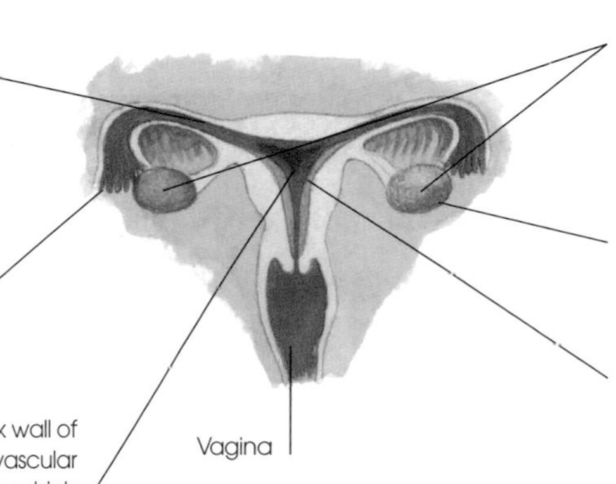

The uterine tube lies folded on the side of the uterus. The ovum may be fertilized here by a spermatozoa.
The fimbriae. Once a month, one ovum is produced. After its release from the ovary it is actively guided by movements of the fimbriae into the uterine tube.
The uterus has a thick wall of smooth muscle and a vascular lining, the endometrium, which undergoes cyclical changes each month, to prepare it for the acceptance of a fertilized ovum.
Vagina
The ovaries are the primary sex organs in the female. They secrete the hormones progesterone and estrogen and produce the female sex cells, the ova.
Take a tea, tincture, or tablet of *Vitex agnus-castus* to regulate the hormones.
A tea of nettles and lady's mantle will help stop heavy bleeding.

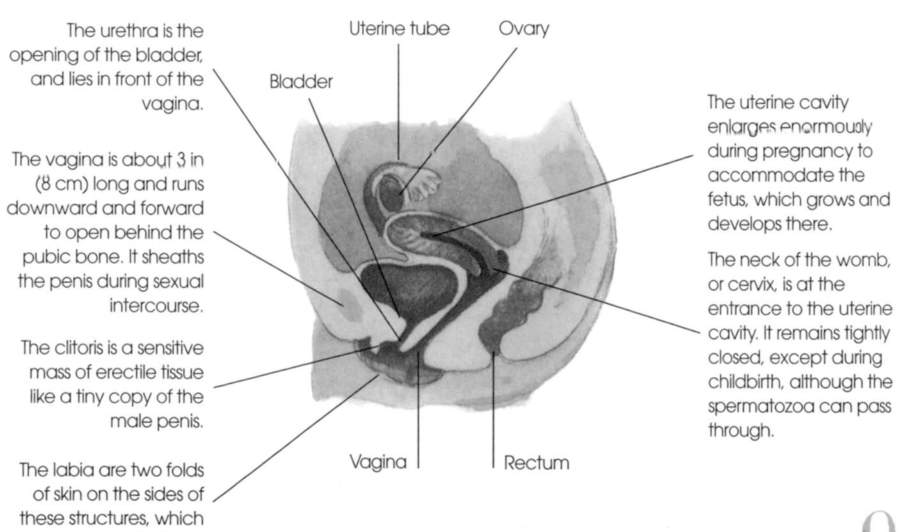

The urethra is the opening of the bladder, and lies in front of the vagina.
The vagina is about 3 in (8 cm) long and runs downward and forward to open behind the pubic bone. It sheaths the penis during sexual intercourse.
The clitoris is a sensitive mass of erectile tissue like a tiny copy of the male penis.
The labia are two folds of skin on the sides of these structures, which hide them.
Uterine tube
Ovary
Bladder
Vagina
Rectum
The uterine cavity enlarges enormously during pregnancy to accommodate the fetus, which grows and develops there.
The neck of the womb, or cervix, is at the entrance to the uterine cavity. It remains tightly closed, except during childbirth, although the spermatozoa can pass through.

The Chinese Medicine Approach

Chinese herbal treatment for menstrual disorders primarily focuses on the blood. Herbs are used to replenish, strengthen, and move the blood, and to stop bleeding. Some prescriptions help after pregnancy, which is seen as a vital time in a woman's life. Many women have complaints in later years, which begin in the postnatal period.

Female Reproductive System Disorders

Premenstrual syndrome (PMS), painful periods, heavy bleeding, endometriosis, and menopausal discomforts are all related to the menstrual cycle. Herbal treatment for these are discussed as well as helpful herbs for conditions related to pregnancy, such as morning sickness, birth, and breastfeeding. Treatment for low fertility and low sex drive will also be given.

Herbal Treatment

Many of the disorders or problems related to the reproductive system are caused by hormone imbalances. There are several herbs which help to regulate hormone activity, such as ginseng, chaste berry (*Vitex agnus-castus*), black cohosh, and wild yam. These will be used along with herbs to strengthen the uterus, nourish the blood, and clear infections. Wild yam contains progesterone, which will help with symptoms of the menopause and postnatal depression.

Right Black cohosh has a balancing effect on hormones, particularly estrogen. It is also used to treat premenstrual syndrome, hormonal imbalances, cramps, and symptoms of the menopause.

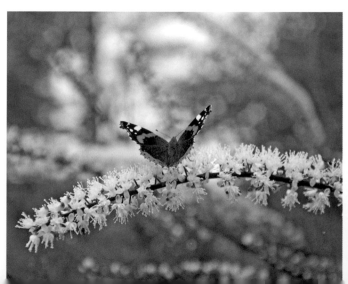

Reproductive Ailments

Premenstrual syndrome (PMS), painful periods, heavy bleeding, endometriosis and menopausal discomforts are all related to the menstrual cycle and herbal treatments for these are discussed in the following pages. Also discussed are treatments for conditions related to pregnancy, low fertility and low sex drive.

Premenstrual Syndrome (PMS)

Irritability, over-sensitivity, lack of coordination, swollen and tender breasts, and water retention are all symptoms of PMS. For some women they are extreme, and can start up to a week before their period is due. The symptoms are generally caused by an excess of the hormone estrogen in relation to progesterone. PMS can also be aggravated by stress and tension in daily life. To help reestablish a hormonal balance, take 20–40 drops (1–2 ml) of *vitex* tincture, or a tablet, before breakfast each morning for several months. For stress and tension, drink a tea of motherwort, skullcap, passionflower, or valerian during the day to help relax.

Below An herbal tea can help alleviate the symptoms of premenstrual tension and aid relaxation.

Water Retention

Use teas or tinctures of dandelion, parsley, or celery seed to clear water retention, which sometimes occurs as a premenstrual syndrome. Reducing the amount of salt in your diet can also help.

Chinese Herbal Treatment The patent formula *Xiao Yao Wan* (Free and Easy Wanderer) is helpful in easing the symptoms of PMS. In Chinese medicine, the liver *qi*, or energy, helps to regulate the flow of the qi and blood in the body. PMS occurs when the *qi* gets "stuck," causing feelings of irritability and frustration, as well as breast tenderness, and bloating. This remedy helps to support the liver so the *qi* flows freely. Take the remedy the week before your period is due.

Dietory Factors Evening primrose oil, taken daily for several months, can help to alleviate PMS. Calcium, magnesium, vitamins E and B-Complex are also helpful, if taken regularly.

Painful Periods

Painful periods cause discomfort that can interrupt work and sleep. For intense cramping pains at the beginning of a period, take a tea or tincture made from crampbark, black cohosh, and licorice (see Herbal Methods chapter, pp.20–47). If it is difficult to sleep with the pain, add valerian and passionflower. Sometimes pain is relieved by a hot bath with relaxing oils or herbs of lavender or rosemary. If pain occurs each month, take *vitex* and/or diet supplements daily to help regulate the hormones.

Chinese Tea Chinese motherwort *(yi mu cao)* helps to encourage bloodflow and regulate menstruation. It is a bitter tea, but helpful when pain is at the onset of bleeding, and eases once the blood flows. It can be prepared on its own as an infusion or with Chinese angelica (*dang gui*) as a Chinese decoction.

Heavy Bleeding

Occasionally, bleeding during a period will be very heavy. Make an infusion using a mixture of lady's mantle, nettles, and raspberry leaf (see Herbal Methods chapter, pp.20–47). The lady's mantle and nettles will help stop the bleeding, and the raspberry leaf strengthens the uterus. If the bleeding is severe or prolonged, consult a doctor for further investigations.

Mugwort (*Moxa*) can be purchased in a *moxa* roll, which is like a cigar. This is lit and held over the abdomen to warm and relax the area, helping to relieve spasms or cramps. Chinese mugwort can be drunk as a tea to help stop prolonged menstrual bleeding when there are feelings of cold and weakness.

Recovery From Periods

Menstruation can leave some women feeling depleted and tired, especially if the bleeding has been heavy. The Chinese patent remedy *Ba Zhen Wan* (Women's Precious Pills, see p.43), is often recommended to restore energy and fortify the blood. It contains the herb Chinese angelica (*dang gui*), which is used as a tonic for the blood.

Delayed or Suppressed Bleeding

The delay or absence of periods can be caused by pregnancy, which should always be checked. Some women have an irregular cycle with no other problems, which may be a natural rhythm for them. Ill-health, emotional upsets, and travel can also affect the menstrual cycle. If periods are irregular in adolescence, it may take time for a cycle to establish itself; try taking 20–40 drops (1–2 ml) of *vitex* each morning for a month. A tea or tincture of *vitex*, with other uterine tonics such as black cohosh and motherwort, taken three times a day, should help to reestablish the menstrual cycle in adult women.

Below Motherwort is a mint with hairy leaves and an intensely bitter taste. It is used to treat premenstrual tension, false labor pains, and to stimulate delayed or suppressed menstruation. It is also known as a mood elevator.

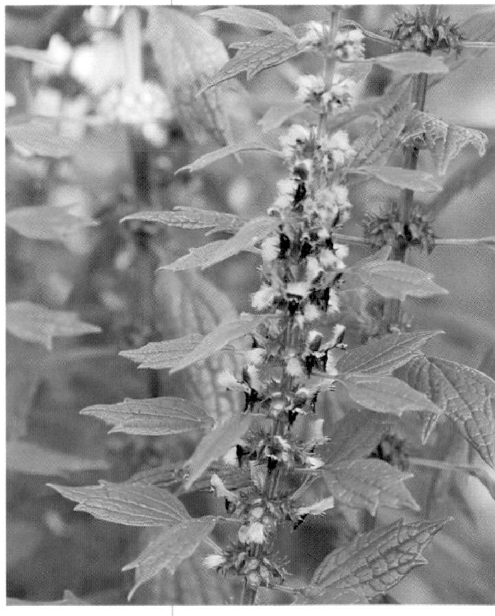

Coming off the Pill

When the contraceptive pill is stopped, the body takes a while to reestablish its natural cycle. Take a mixture of *vitex*, black cohosh, licorice, and motherwort in equal parts as a tea three times a day for the first two weeks after stopping the pill. Drink this twice a day for the third week, and once a day for the fourth week.

Endometriosis

This is a painful condition in which the uterine lining "escapes" from the uterus into other areas in the pelvis. Endometriosis fluctuates with hormonal changes, causing pain and sometimes very heavy bleeding. To help rebalance the hormones, take *vitex*. Use a combination of crampbark, lady's mantle, and nettles to help ease pain and stop heavy bleeding. There are other helpful herbs, but these should only be prescribed by a medical herbalist.

Massage Oil Massage oils of either lavender, rosemary, or camomile on to the abdomen to relieve cramping pain. Put finely chopped pieces of the herb in vegetable oil. Place this in the sun or a warm place for two weeks. Strain the herbs from the liquid using a fine piece of muslin. Store the oil in a dark glass container (see Herbal Methods chapter, pp.20–47).

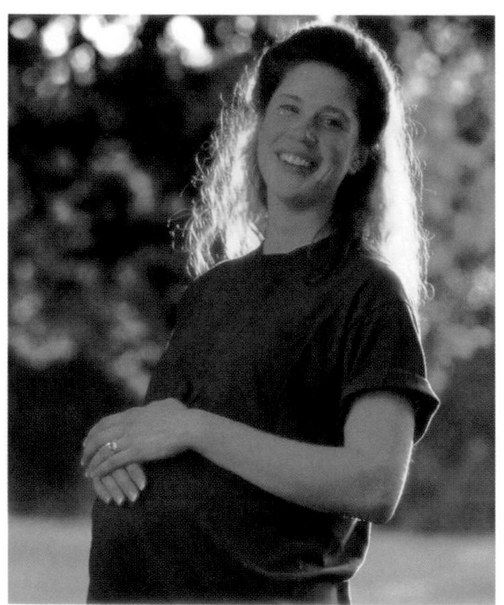

Above Herbs can provide an effective and safe treatment for minor complaints of pregnancy, such as morning sickness.

Pregnancy

Pregnancy is a very special time in a woman's life. Herbal remedies have been used for centuries to help women through pregnancy and childbirth.

Many herbs are safe to use and very effective; however, some herbs should be avoided (see below).

Herbs to Avoid Some herbs have a stimulating effect on the uterus and should be avoided during pregnancy. Here is a list of common herbs which should not be used: aloe vera, barberry, coltsfoot, comfrey, goldenseal, juniper, male fern, pennyroyal, pokeroot, rue, sage, tansy, thuja, and wormwood. If you have any doubts about using a herb in pregnancy, please check with a qualified herbalist.

Threatened Miscarriage

Miscarriage is often the body's natural response to a pregnancy that is not right from the start, and no amount of herbal intervention will stop this. However, if a woman is under stress, or her diet is inadequate, herbs can help to strengthen and nourish her, which may prevent a threatened miscarriage. Make a decoction using herbs to tone the uterus and relax spasms. Use a mixture of false unicorn root with one-half part crampbark in 1½ pints (800 ml) water. Simmer gently for 10 minutes and drink 8 fl oz (200 ml) three times a day. Add skullcap or valerian if there is stress.

Chinese Herbal Treatment Perilla leaf *(zi su ye)* is a warm and aromatic herb that can be taken for threatened miscarriage and/or morning sickness. Place ¼ oz (6 g) of the dried herb in 8 fl oz (200 ml) of water. Simmer for 15 minutes, then strain and drink twice a day. For morning sickness, add ⅕ oz (4 g) dried orange peel (*chen pi*) before cooking to help ease nausea.

Morning Sickness

Many women experience morning sickness and nausea during the first few months of pregnancy. It is often caused by hormonal changes and low blood sugar, so its symptoms are often strongest in the morning. Drink a sweet tea of meadowsweet, camomile, or peppermint before getting up. Ginger, in the form of a biscuit, capsule, or tea, may also help settle the stomach. Drink these teas throughout the day as needed. In North America raspberry leaf tea is sometimes taken for nausea in pregnancy. However, in the UK it is not used until the last three months of pregnancy (see labor, below).

Labor

During the last three months of pregnancy, drink herbal teas of raspberry leaves or squaw vine to help strengthen the uterus and prepare it for childbirth. Drink 1 pint (600 ml) of tea a day. While in labor, if contractions are weak and ineffective, drink a tea made from a mixture of raspberry leaves and black cohosh with a slice of ginger. If pains are very sharp and cramping, add crampbark. Massage the back and legs with dilute oils of lavender or camomile.

Recovery from Childbirth

For many women childbirth is not an easy process, and may leave feelings of exhaustion and depletion. An herbal remedy that is often used in China is a decoction made from Chinese angelica (*dang gui)* and astragalus (*huang qi*). The angelica revitalizes the blood and the astragalus strengthens the *qi*, or energy. It is especially helpful if there has been a large loss of blood or a long labor. Use 1½ oz (30 g) astragalus and ¼ oz (6 g) Chinese angelica in 1½ pints (800 ml) water. Simmer for one hour. Strain and drink warm throughout the day. Take daily until strength and vitality return.

Breastfeeding

Whenever possible, breastfeeding is the best way to ensure the child receives the right nutrients and immunity. To increase the flow of milk, drink a tea of fennel seed in combination with nettles, vervain, or

Below Breastfeeding ensures a baby receives the right nutrients and immunity. A tea of fennel seeds will encourage the milk flow

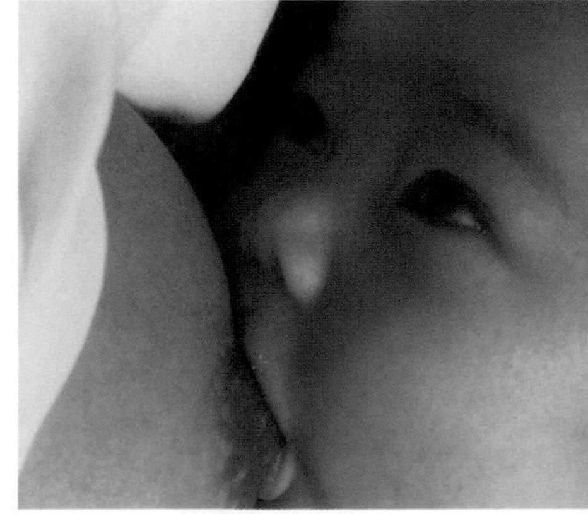

borage. Encourage the baby to suck as much as possible, making sure that the mother is relaxed and rested.

Painful Breasts

When the milk flow becomes obstructed, the breasts can become enlarged and engorged. This can be very uncomfortable and may lead to mastitis, an infection of the milk glands. It is important to keep the baby feeding, although this may be uncomfortable. Apply ice-cold compresses made from pokeroot tea to the breasts, or use water with a few drops of lavender, fennel, or geranium oils. Place fresh cabbage leaves or rhubarb leaves in the bra between feeds. For sore, cracked nipples, use ointments of marigold (calendula) or chickweed, or rub a drop of breastmilk into the nipple after the feed.

Mastitis

If mastitis does set in, take a tea or tincture made from echinacea, dandelion root, yarrow, and a small amount of pokeroot. The echinacea and dandelion root will help to clear the infection, the yarrow will relieve any fever, and the pokeroot will help to clear the milk ducts. Drink this three times a day until the condition clears. Apply a warm poultice of either slippery elm and marshmallow or comfrey to the breasts (see Herbal Methods chapter, pp.20–47). Bathing the breasts in hot water and warm compresses of distilled witch hazel will also relieve discomfort.

Menopause

The menopause is a normal time of change and transition in a woman's life. The first signs may be changes in the menstrual cycle, with periods becoming irregular, and hot flashes. Other discomforts may include mood swings, depression, irritability, insomnia, joint pain, low sex drive, and tiredness. For many women, emotional issues such as aging, children leaving home, and career decisions increase the pressure to reevaluate their lives. It may be difficult to separate the changes in their life from the changes in their body. A holistic approach can be supportive emotionally and physically.

Hot Flashes

Hot flashes are a common symptom of the menopause. To relieve them, use a tea of sage and motherwort. Take vitamin E and evening primrose oil daily. Black cohosh (see Herbal Directory, pp.164–215) is also useful in the treatment of symptoms of the menopause.

Tiredness and Depression

Drink a tea made from St. John's wort, skullcap, or vervain. Try to avoid having caffeine, substituting relaxing and refreshing herbal teas, such as lime blossom, rosemary, and lemon balm. Take a good multivitamin and mineral daily.

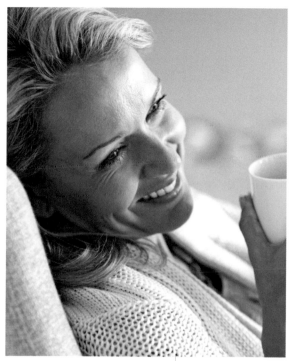

Above During the menopause, try an herbal solution to ease discomforts such as hot flushes, depression, joint pains, and insomnia. Use the herbs over a period of time to help reestablish a hormonal balance.

Herbal Treatment A mixture of the following herbs will help the body to adapt to the changes in hormones, and to establish a new level of functioning. Use a combination of *vitex*, false unicorn root, St. John's wort, angelica (*dang gui*), and motherwort for several months until discomfort is eased. Use 1 oz (20 g) of the mixture with 1½ pints (800 ml) water. Prepare the angelica and false unicorn root as a decoction, simmering for 30 minutes, then adding the *vitex*, St. John's wort, and motherwort. Drink this throughout the day (see Herbal Methods chapter, pp.20–47).

Joint Pains

A traditional Chinese herbal remedy to ease joint pains and cramping can be made from lycium fruit (*gou qi zi*) and licorice (*gan cao*). This helps to strengthen the circulation and nourish the blood. It may also help dry skin and dryness of the eyes. Prepare as a Chinese herbal

Opposite The female reproductive system can benefit from camomile due to the plant's capacity to soothe uterine spasms, and induce menstruation. Drinking camomile tea has been found to be beneficial in treating PMS and menstrual cramps.

decoction using 1 oz (20 g) lycium fruit and ½ oz (10 g) of licorice in 1½ pints (800 ml) of water. Simmer for 30 minutes. Strain and drink one half in the morning and one half in the evening.

Low Sex Drive in Women

Low sex drive can have several causes, such as general tiredness and depression, frustration in a relationship, or hormonal imbalance. It is important to understand the cause so that treatment can be effective. Herbal treatment will help with tiredness and hormonal balance, but counseling will be more effective if there is a problem in the relationship. To help balance the hormones, take 20–40 drops (1–2 ml) of *vitex* tincture each morning. Make a Chinese herbal decoction using Chinese angelica (*dang gui*) and licorice (*gan cao*) to help overcome feelings of weakness. Drink teas of camomile, vervain, and skullcap to help relax and ease tensions. Use oils of rose, neroli, geranium, and jasmine in an herbal bath or a massage oil.

Impotence

A tea of damiana and saw palmetto berries will help to boost the male hormones. Add licorice, cinnamon, and ginger to warm and strengthen the body. Use oils of frankincense and cinnamon in a bath or massage. Take regular decoctions of ginseng (see Herbal Methods chapter, pp.20–47), for no longer than three months, to help relieve general tiredness and revitalize sexual energy. Gingko will increase the blood supply to the penis. Relaxation, visualization, and sometimes therapy are needed to deal with psychological impotence or performance anxiety.

Infertility

For many couples, difficulty in conceiving can have an enormous effect on the rest of their lives. Many tests can be carried out to help find the source of the problem; medical treatment can be risky and very expensive. If there are no obvious structural problems, such as ovarian cysts or blocked fallopian tubes, it is worth trying herbal treatment because it helps to stimulate the body to heal itself. If the suggestions here do not help, try seeing a medical herbalist for a private consultation.

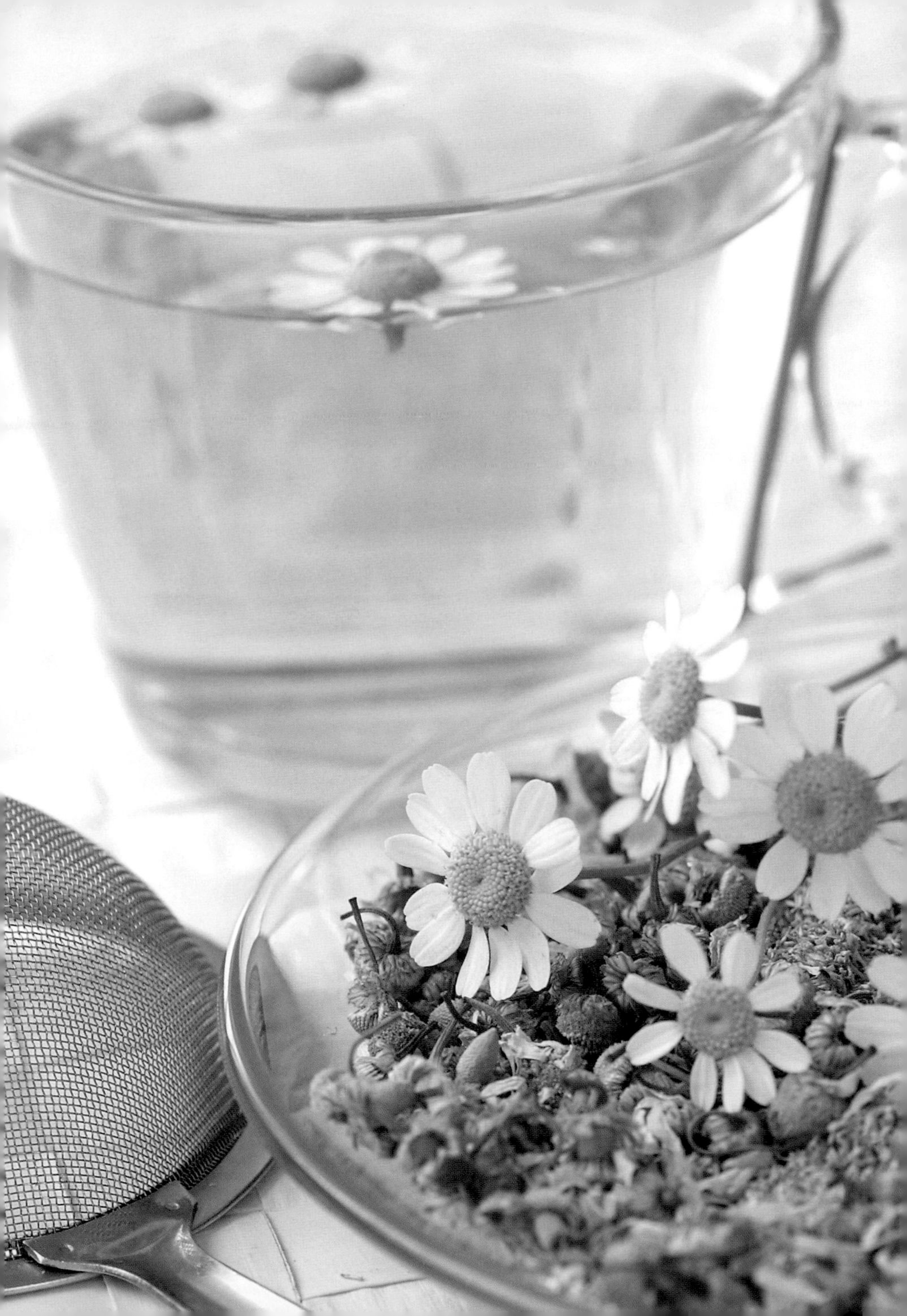

Low Sperm Count

A healthy diet, free from junk food (such as ready meals), and avoiding alcohol, cigarettes, and caffeine will help to increase the number of healthy sperm. Avoid wearing tight clothing and having hot baths. Take a combination of damiana, saw palmetto, celery seeds, licorice, and ginger as a tea or a tincture on a regular basis (see Herbal Methods section, pp.20–47). Drink ginseng as a Chinese decoction or as a medicinal brandy (see below), except in cases of high blood pressure.

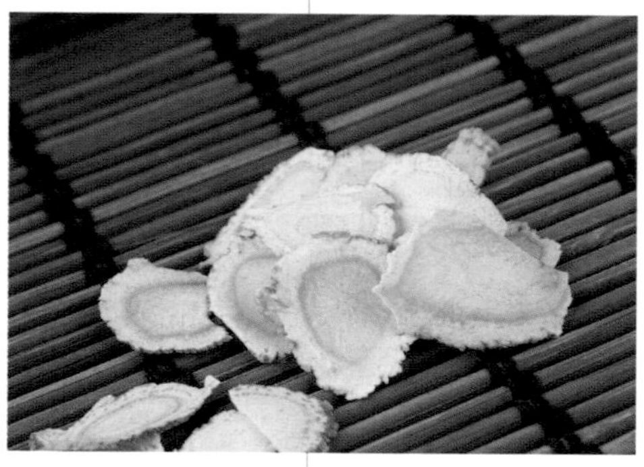

Above Ginseng root is thought to have various benefits to female fertility. Peruvian ginseng may increase egg follicle development, while Panax ginseng is believed to act as a reproductive tonic through its adaptogenic properties.

Difficulty Conceiving

These herbs help to balance a woman's hormones and nourish the blood and uterus, so they will help to encourage conception in cases where there is no known cause for difficulty. Over several months, drink a tea of *vitex*, false unicorn root, roses, nettles, and marigold. Supplements of evening primrose oil, kelp, royal jelly, and vitamin B may also help.

Ginseng Medicinal Brandy Take 4 oz (100 g) of good-quality ginseng root and place it in a bottle with 2 pints (1 liter) brandy. Soak for two to three weeks. Drink approximately 1½ tsp (6 ml) a day to help restore vitality and strengthen the body. Avoid using ginseng if there is high blood pressure. It should not be used during pregnancy.

The Male Reproductive System

The primary sex organs in the male are the two testes. As they need to be kept cool, they lie in the scrotum outside the body.

Erection of the penis is caused by arterial dilatation controlled by the parasympathetic nervous system. The spongy spaces in the corpora become filled with blood at full arterial pressure.

Ejaculation expels just over half a teaspoon of semen, containing about 300 million spermatozoa, into the female genital tract during sexual intercourse.

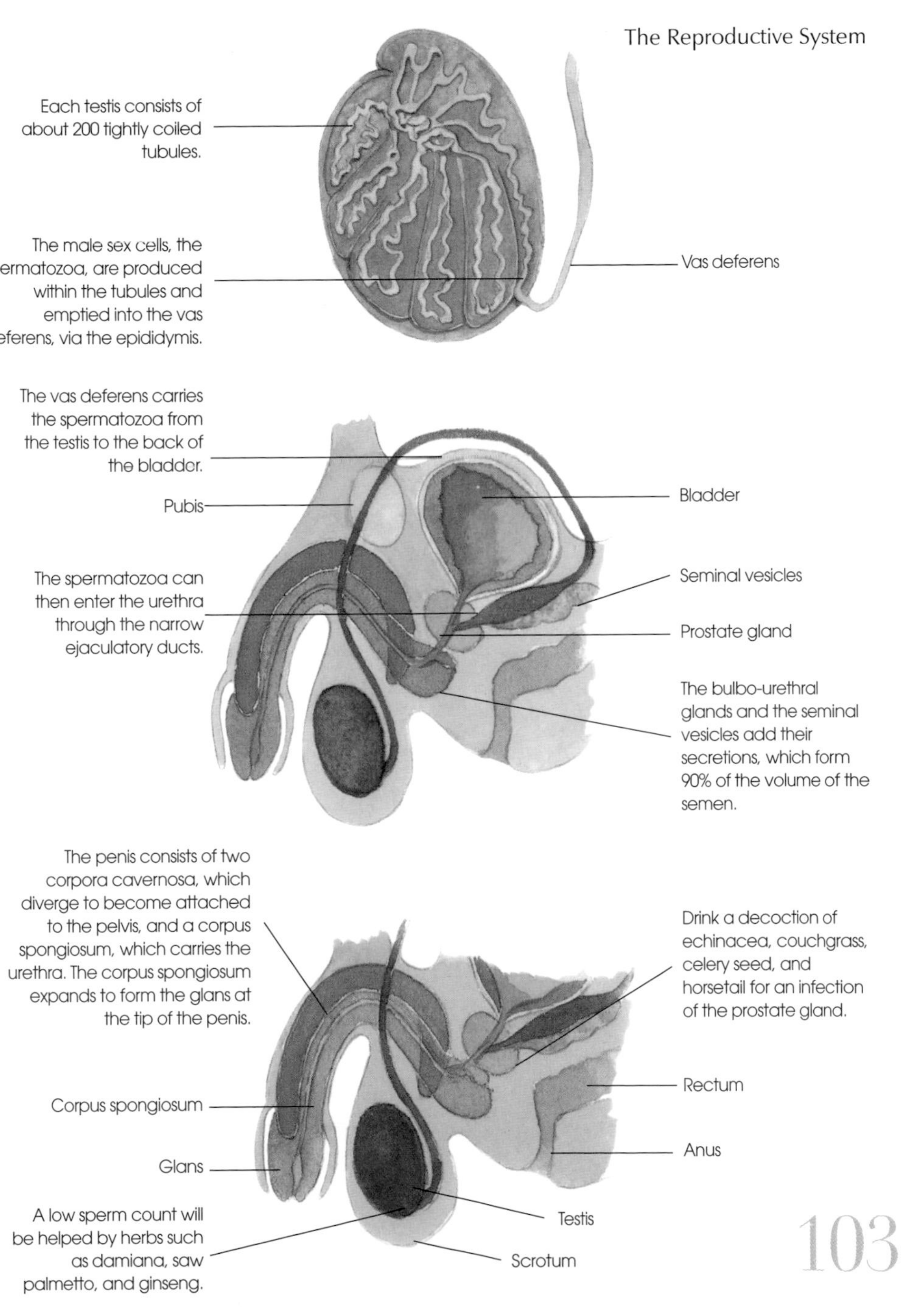
Each testis consists of about 200 tightly coiled tubules.
The male sex cells, the spermatozoa, are produced within the tubules and emptied into the vas deferens, via the epididymis.
Vas deferens
The vas deferens carries the spermatozoa from the testis to the back of the bladder.
Pubis
Bladder
The spermatozoa can then enter the urethra through the narrow ejaculatory ducts.
Seminal vesicles
Prostate gland
The bulbo-urethral glands and the seminal vesicles add their secretions, which form 90% of the volume of the semen.
The penis consists of two corpora cavernosa, which diverge to become attached to the pelvis, and a corpus spongiosum, which carries the urethra. The corpus spongiosum expands to form the glans at the tip of the penis.
Drink a decoction of echinacea, couchgrass, celery seed, and horsetail for an infection of the prostate gland.
Rectum
Corpus spongiosum
Anus
Glans
Testis
A low sperm count will be helped by herbs such as damiana, saw palmetto, and ginseng.
Scrotum

The Endocrine System

The endocrine, or glandular, system controls and balances the production of hormones, which have a profound effect on the state of health of the body. The hypothalamus of the brain, and the pituitary, thyroid, and adrenal glands, the pancreas, testes, and ovaries are all parts of this system.

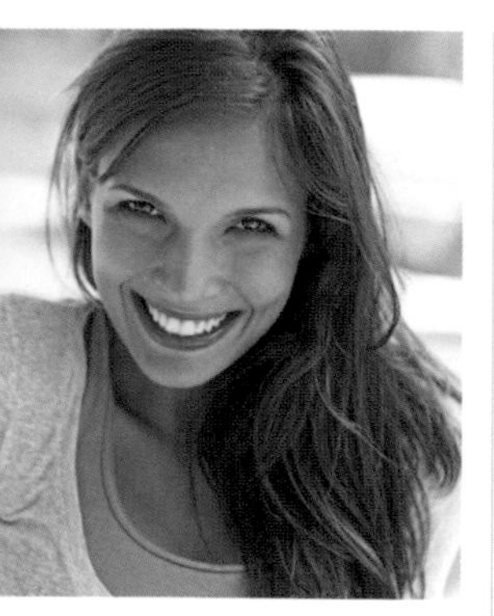

Above A well-functioning endocrine system secretes endorphins such as seratonin which can boost our happiness and well-being.

The processes of the endocrine system are too complex to explain in detail here. Basically, the endocrine system secretes hormones into the bloodstream, which act as chemical messengers that travel to all parts of the body. Hormone production in many cases is controlled by a negative feedback system: an over-production of one hormone will sometimes cause a decrease in another, until the balance in the body is restored. The pituitary gland plays a central role in maintaining this harmony or homeostasis.

Interaction with the Body

The effects of the endocrine system can be felt in all parts of the body. It has a strong connection with the nervous system and our emotions. For example, the adrenal glands will produce more adrenaline in dangerous situations. This will then encourage the heart to beat faster so that blood gets to the muscles to encourage their rapid movements, along with feelings of fear and excitement. The sexual hormones in the testes and ovaries are responsible for the reproductive process, and have a strong connection to romantic feelings. The hormones secreted by the thyroid and pancreas affect our metabolism and blood sugar levels. The functioning of these glands will also alter our moods and state of mind.

The Chinese Medicine Approach

According to traditional Chinese medicine, the endocrine system is not related to just one system. Treatment is according to individual symptoms, as well as information obtained from the pulse and tongue. Generally, the functioning of the adrenal glands is treated specifically with herbs that support it, such as licorice (*gan cao*), or ginseng, if there are symptoms of tiredness and depletion. Various seaweeds are added to prescriptions to regulate the thyroid.

How the Endocrine System Works

For the widespread activities of the body, such as growth, metabolism, water/salt balance, and reproduction, which do not demand rapid changes, coordination throughout the body is affected by chemical messengers. These are the hormones produced by the ductless endocrine glands.

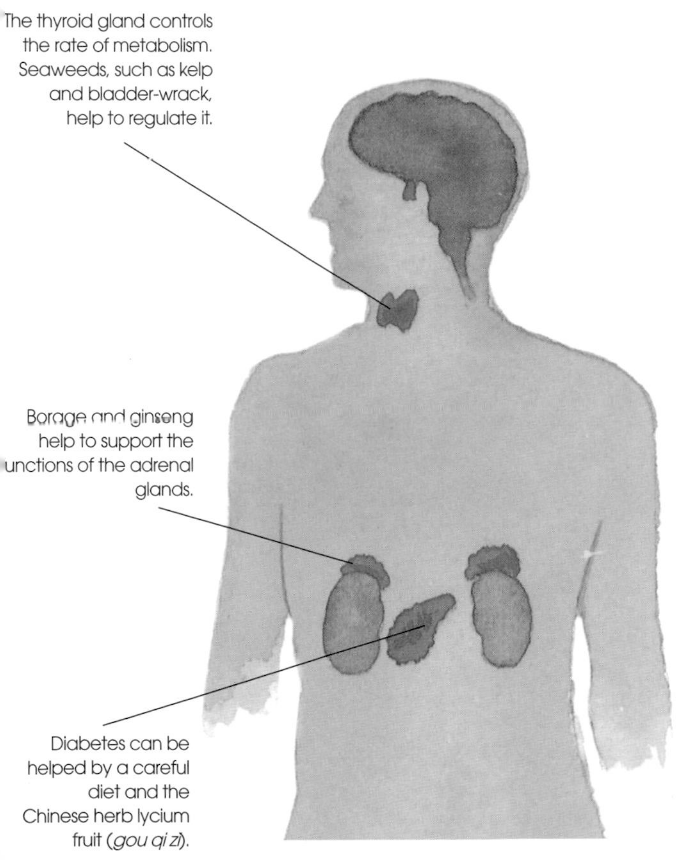

The thyroid gland controls the rate of metabolism. Seaweeds, such as kelp and bladder-wrack, help to regulate it.
Borage and ginseng help to support the unctions of the adrenal glands.
Diabetes can be helped by a careful diet and the Chinese herb lycium fruit (*gou qi zi*).

Left Glands in the body. Ovaries and testes are also part of the endocrine system, although their primary purpose is to produce gametes (egg and sporm.)

Below Artichokes are said to affect blood sugar and insulin levels. A medium-sized artichoke has ¼ oz (6 g) of dietary fiber. As an additional benefit, fiber helps to keep your blood sugar stable.

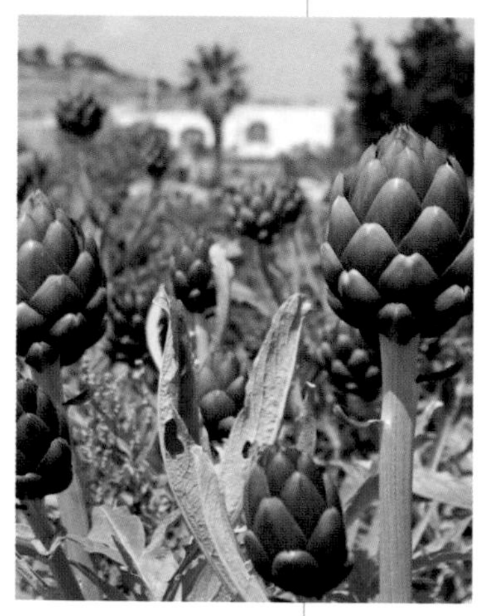

Ailments of the Endocrine System

In this section, treatments for diabetes, overactive thyroid, underactive thyroid, and the adrenal glands are discussed. Suggestions for treatments for the ailments related to the testes and ovaries may be found in the section related to the reproductive system (see pp.90–103). If stress or nervous exhaustion are part of the symptom picture, consult the section on the nervous system (see pp.144–157).

The Pancreas

The pancreas is a large gland that secretes the digestive enzymes which break down protein, fat, and carbohydrates. It also produces insulin and glucagon, which regulate the amount of sugar in the blood.

Diabetes Mellitus

Diabetes occurs when the pancreas—or, more specifically, the islets of Langerhans, which are part of it—malfunctions and does not produce enough insulin. Blood sugar levels are higher than normal, and extra doses of insulin may need to be taken, either via a syringe or tablets, depending on the severity of the diabetes. In milder cases, usually occurring in people over the age of fifty, a diet which avoids sugars and controls carbohydrate intake may be adequate to normalize the blood sugar levels. Professional advice is needed for herbal treatments. There are records of herbs and foods such as allspice, artichoke, banana, burdock, cabbage, carrot, ginseng, nettles, oats, olives, onion, papaya, peas, spinach, sunflower, and turnip having properties that help to reduce the blood sugar level. The Chinese herb, lycium fruit (*gou qi zi),* can be eaten daily as a treatment for diabetes.

The Thyroid

The thyroid gland secretes hormones which help to regulate the metabolism of the body. They have an effect on the rate of digestion, appetite, weight gain or loss, and general feelings of anxiety, depression, and tiredness.

Underactive Thyroid

In this condition, the body's basic rate of activity is lowered causing symptoms of weight gain, apathy, and depression. Herbal treatment consists of nervine tonics and a specific plant that has an action on the thyroid, called bladderwrack, which is a type of seaweed. Combine two parts of bladderwrack with one part of damiana, nettles, and oats. Drink 8 fl oz (200 ml), three times a day. Take plenty of gentle exercise, such as yoga or t'ai chi, to help stimulate and keep energy moving.

Overactive Thyroid

This is the opposite of the condition above, where there is an overproduction of thyroid hormones. Symptoms include overactivity,

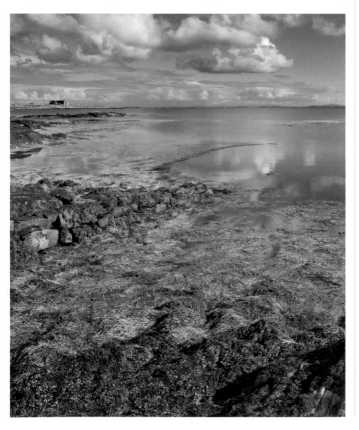

Left Kelp and bladderwrack are two types of seaweed which help to regulate the function of the thyroid gland. Take these in combination with other herbs.

Facing page Take time to relax and enjoy life since long-term stress and strain can undermine the balancing functions of the thyroid, pancreas, and adrenal glands.

with restlessness, anxiety, tension, and weight loss. Take a combination of nervine relaxants with kelp for an over-active thyroid. A helpful combination would be two parts of kelp to one part each of nettles, valerian, and yarrow.

The Adrenal Glands

The adrenal glands are located just above the kidneys and secrete the hormone adrenaline. In stressful situations, adrenaline is released into the bloodstream to prepare the body for fight-or-flight by increasing the heart rate, raising blood pressure, and stimulating breathing. Long-term stressful situations are sure to exhaust the body and deplete the adrenal glands.

Herbal Treatment There are several herbs which support the function of the adrenal glands. Borage and ginseng are beneficial in long-term stressful situations. Take them as teas or tinctures to help build up the adrenal glands and revitalize the body. Licorice or Chinese licorice (*gan cao*) is also used as a tonic for the adrenal glands, and is especially helpful for recovering from the side-effects of steroid drugs.

Right Licorice slows down the breakdown of adrenal hormones in the body, helping to maintain them at optimal levels.

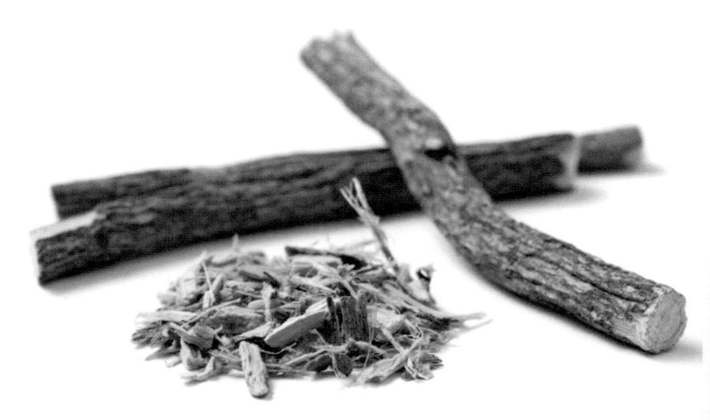

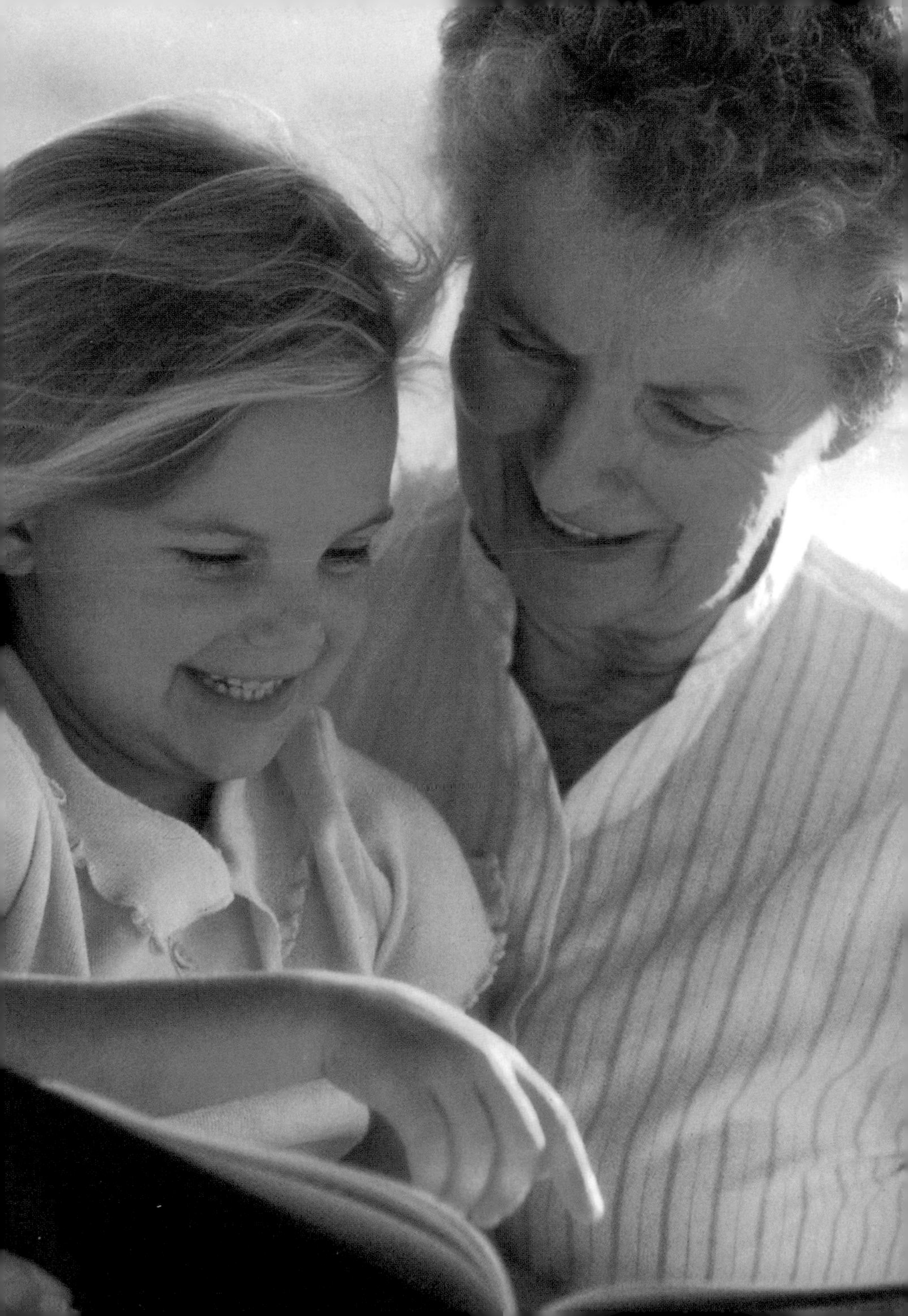

The Skin

The skin is the body's largest organ, completely encasing the other organs and tissues. Its many functions include protection, excretion, and sensory perception. Ailments are rarely symptomatic of the skin itself; more often they are signs of complex processes involving aspects of the whole body.

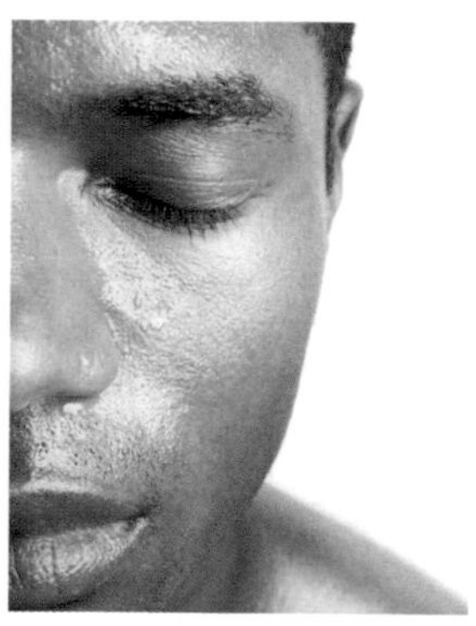

Above Because it is in contact with the environment, skin plays a key role in protecting the body from pathogens and excessive water loss.

The skin comprises two layers: the epidermis and the dermis. The epidermis is the outer layer and has four or five layers, with more on the soles of the feet and palms of the hands. The dermis is the innermost layer, containing the blood vessels, nerves, glands, and hair follicles. There are two types of glands in the skin. The sebaceous glands secrete an oil to keep the skin soft and supple. The sudoriferous, or sweat, glands pass through the dermis and open as a pore through which salts, water, and acids are excreted as perspiration.

Interaction with the Body

The skin is responsible for excreting about one-quarter of the body's wastes. Any problem with the skin puts a strain on the other three major organs involved in eliminating wastes: the kidneys, lungs, and bowels. Any dysfunction with these organs will also have an effect on the skin. The skin helps to regulate body temperature through perspiration, which acts as a cooling process. It protects the more vital organs from extremes in temperature, harmful rays from the sun, and invasive microorganisms.

The Chinese Medicine Approach

Traditional Chinese medicine sees the skin as the outer lung, which helps to explain the high correlation between asthma and eczema in many children. Chinese herbs are particularly good for skin conditions. Many herbs used to treat the skin are used to help other organs to function more efficiently. Often the diagnosis is based on the appearance of the skin, as well as other, traditional, techniques. A bright-red rash that bleeds easily will be due to too much heat; a weeping skin will be caused by excessive dampness; and dry, brittle skin will indicate a lack of moisture. The herbs used will heal the whole body by clearing or tonifying, depending on the needs of the individual. Changes in the skin condition as it heals will need different herbal prescriptions. It is advisable, therefore, to have an individual consultation with a traditional Chinese herbalist.

How the Skin Works

The skin is sensitive to a variety of stimuli. Its sensitivity varies from place to place on the body. The fingertips and face are very sensitive; the skin of the back is least sensitive.

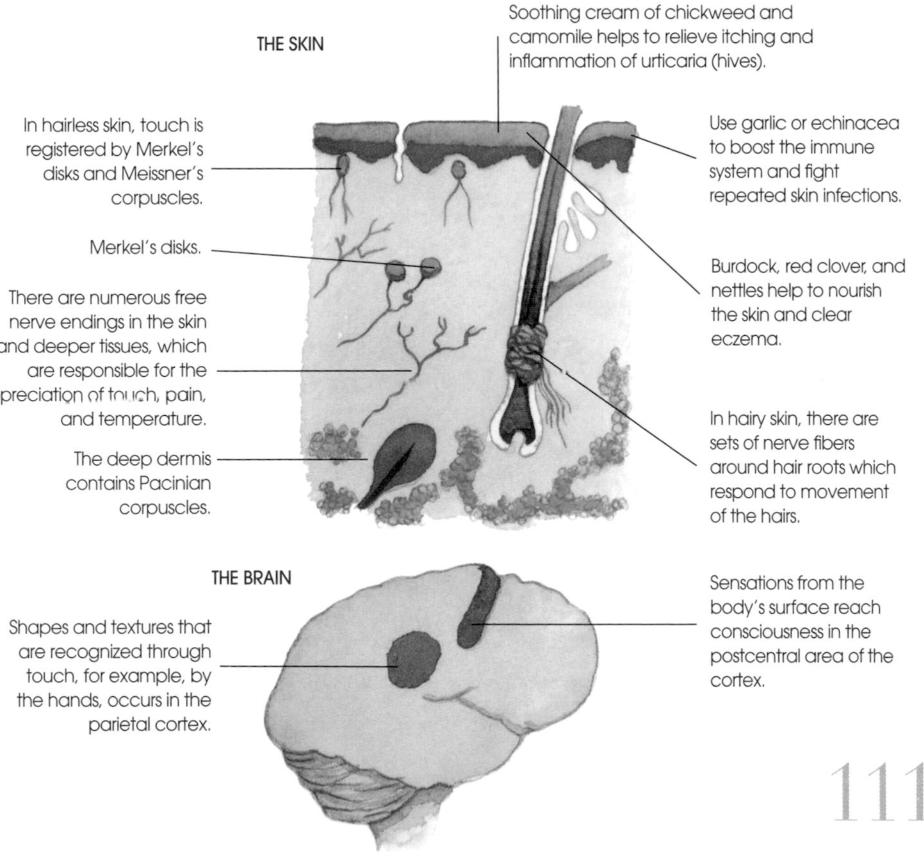

THE SKIN
Soothing cream of chickweed and camomile helps to relieve itching and inflammation of urticaria (hives).
In hairless skin, touch is registered by Merkel's disks and Meissner's corpuscles.
Use garlic or echinacea to boost the immune system and fight repeated skin infections.
Merkel's disks.
Burdock, red clover, and nettles help to nourish the skin and clear eczema.
There are numerous free nerve endings in the skin and deeper tissues, which are responsible for the appreciation of touch, pain, and temperature.
In hairy skin, there are sets of nerve fibers around hair roots which respond to movement of the hairs.
The deep dermis contains Pacinian corpuscles.
THE BRAIN
Sensations from the body's surface reach consciousness in the postcentral area of the cortex.
Shapes and textures that are recognized through touch, for example, by the hands, occurs in the parietal cortex.

Prevention of Skin Disease

There are many different types of skin disease, which means there are many causes. It is difficult to generalize because what may work for one person does not necessarily work for others. Some skin conditions indicate an inherited tendency, such as eczema and psoriasis. Others, such as acne, may be worse at certain times in a person's life. Each skin condition will need specific advice for treatment and prevention. A good diet, containing fresh fruit and vegetables, and drinking plenty of fresh water, taking brisk exercise, breathing fresh air, and cultivating a peaceful state of mind will all help the quality of the skin, and the quality of life itself.

Skin Ailments

Skin problems vary enormously, from those that are chronic, such as eczema and psoriasis, to those which might be a fleeting allergic reaction, such as a rash or urticaria (hives). Bacterial, viral, and fungal infections may cause acne, boils, warts, herpes, and athlete's foot. These conditions are all covered in this section, along with external skin problems such as bruises, burns, and wounds.

Eczema

Eczema is an itchy skin condition which has various forms and stages. It can appear as a red, itchy rash or weepy blisters, which then change to dry, cracked skin as healing takes place. Longstanding eczma can appear as dry, scaly, hard, thickened skin. If the skin is broken by scratching, it can become infected and create further inflammation. Eczema may have many causes, and it is important to find out what may help and what may aggravate it. Try to wear cotton clothing. Use a pure soap and laundry detergent for sensitive skins. Water, especially if it is very chlorinated, can dry the skin, so use oil in the bath and moisturizing creams afterward. Avoid scratching by wearing light cotton clothing that covers itchy areas. Eczema may be aggravated by animals or hayfever. If stress is a factor, try to deal with contributory factors and find a more relaxing way of life.

Dietary Factors Eczema can be triggered by food allergies, particularly dairy produce, eggs, and wheat. Other foods which can

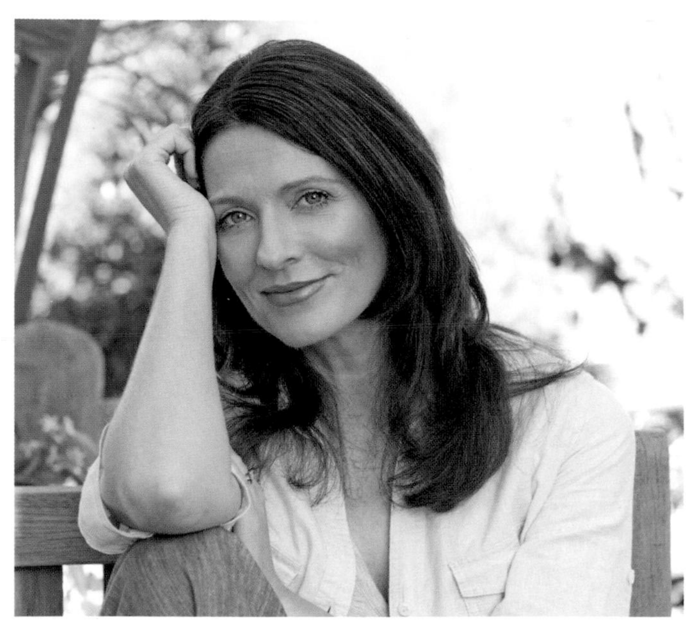

Left Eating a good diet and drinking lots of water will help to keep the skin clear of blemishes.

cause skin reactions are tomatoes, citrus fruits, sugar, chocolate, pork, beef, peppers, and eggplant (aubergine). To find out if the person has a food sensitivity, eliminate one of these foods for ten days, then introduce it back into the diet and observe whether there is any reaction. There may be nutritional deficiencies, and supplements of evening primrose oil, vitamins A, B, C, and E, and the minerals zinc, magnesium, calcium, and iron may help.

Herbal Treatment A hot herbal tea of echinacea and yarrow will help cleanse the blood and support the immune system. Add borage or licorice to support the adrenal glands, especially if steroid creams have been used or are being reduced. Burdock, red clover, and nettles will help to cleanse and nourish the skin. Make a decoction of several herbs and drink 1 pint (600 ml) a day. Externally, use a few drops of camomile or lemon balm oil to soothe dry skin. Aloe vera gel or comfrey ointment are also helpful. If the eczema is infected, try a bath with lavender oil, sea salt, or cider vinegar. Use a compress of marigold, burdock, or yellow dock on the infected area.

Psoriasis

Psoriasis is an extremely common skin condition. It is distressing because of its appearance: red areas, often raised and clearly marked, produce excess epidermis, which can itch and flake off. Psoriasis often clears up with the help of exposure to sunshine and seawater. However, stress, food allergies, and nutritional deficiencies can aggravate it in a similar way to eczema.

Herbal Treatment Take herbal teas or tinctures to help relax and strengthen the nervous system. Camomile, skullcap, vervain, and lemon balm are all nervine tonics, and can be taken on a daily basis. Use motherwort or lime blossom if there are high blood pressure or palpitations. An infusion or decoction of burdock, nettles, cleavers, and yellow dock will help to cleanse and nourish the body (see Herbal Methods section pp.20–47). If the condition has not cleared up after three months, consult a professional herbalist.

Acne

Acne tends to be related to hormonal changes that occur during adolescence or around the time of the menopause. Diet can also play an important role. Make a serious attempt to avoid fatty foods, dairy produce, chocolate, alcohol, sweets, tea, and coffee; eat plenty of fresh fruits and vegetables. Take an herbal tea made from a combination of dandelion root, burdock, cleavers, and echinacea to cleanse the blood. To help regulate hormonal imbalance, women can take chaste berry (*Vitex agnus castus*) daily. Steam your face for five to ten minutes to clean the pores with hot infusions of lavender, camomile, or thyme. Rinse your face with rosewater, honeywater, or a dilute infusion of marigold tea to tone and close the pores. Do this every day until the skin heals (this may take several months).

Urticaria (Hives)

Urticaria is an allergic skin reaction which appears as a red rash. Sometimes the reaction can affect the mouth and lips, and in these cases a doctor should be called immediately because serious breathing difficulties could occur. It is important to identify the allergen, which is usually a food, perfume, an insect sting, or even strong sunlight.

Herbal Bath and Compress To relieve itching and inflammation in acute reactions, make a strong infusion of burdock or chickweed and pour it into a hot bath and soak the body thoroughly, or make a compress from a strong decoction of burdock root and yellow dock.

Soothing Cream Use a combination of chickweed and camomile to make a cream to relieve itching and inflammation (see Herbal Methods section, pp.20–47). The chickweed is cooling, and the camomile helps to calm and soothe the irritation of the skin.

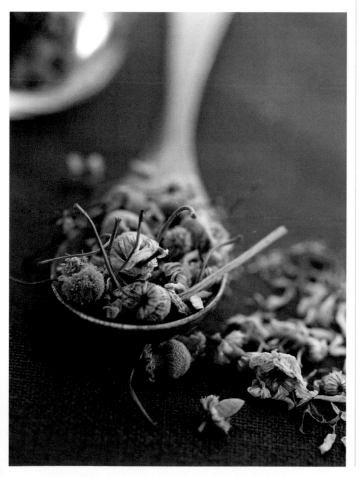

Left A bath of camomile, burdock, or chickweed will help to relieve acute urticaria.

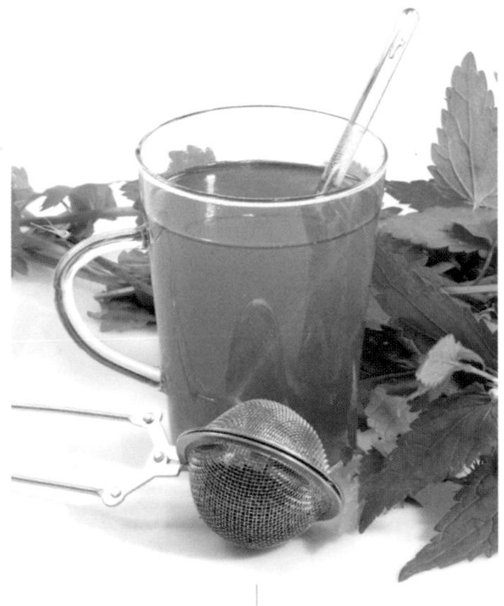

Abscesses and Boils

Abscesses and boils are eruptions of the skin that are infected with pus. They occur when the skin becomes infected with the *Staphylococcus pyogenes* bacteria, often because the body is under stress or weakened. To heal these skin ailments, both internal and external treatments are needed. Use herbs to boost the immune system, such as echinacea and garlic. Drink a mixture of burdock, nettles, and pokeroot to help resolve the infection. Repeated attacks of boils can indicate that the body is run down and in need of rest and relaxation. Contact your doctor if the boils do not come to a head in a few days, or if there is a fever.

Above The nettle plant is a panacea when taken internally, and it can also be used to treat external disorders such as skin conditions, bleeding and wounds.

External Treatment There are several different types of compress and poultice to help bring out pus and discharge. You can apply these for an hour or so, three times a day. Make a poultice of slippery elm and marshmallow leaves, and apply this as hot as possible (see Herbal Methods section, pp.20–47). Burdock, comfrey, or Chinese dandelion (*pu gong ying*) can also be mashed in hot water and used in a similar manner to make a poultice to draw out the infection.

Cabbage-Leaf Poultice Take a few of the inner leaves of a white cabbage and wash them well. Remove the large ribs. Tap the leaves with a rolling pin to soften them, and place them directly onto the infection. Hold them in place with a bandage for half an hour. Remove them and replace with new leaves.

Warts

Warts are caused by a viral infection, and can only take root if the body is susceptible or vulnerable. Treatment needs to be both internal and external. Drink teas of cleavers, pokeroot, and prickly ash to clear the lymphatic system and strengthen the body. Externally, apply a tincture of the herb thuja (*Thuja occidentalis*) twice a day for a month. Vitamin E oil or garlic oil can also be put on the warts to help clear them up.

Herpes Simplex or Cold Sores

This is another common viral infection that usually takes hold in the body early in life. The infection remains unnoticed until the resistance in the body is lowered. Cold sores can be triggered by various factors, such as other infections, menstruation, stress, or poor diet. Treatment includes boosting the immune system by taking high doses of vitamin C ½ tsp (1 g) daily, and improving diet and lifestyle. Make a decoction of echinacea, cleavers, oats, and pokeroot to help clear the lymphatic system (see Herbal Methods section, pp.20–47). Drink the tea twice a day for two weeks. Externally, apply a lotion made from echinacea and myrrh. A commercially produced extract of *Melissa officinalis* applied topically is also helpful in the treatment of cold sores.

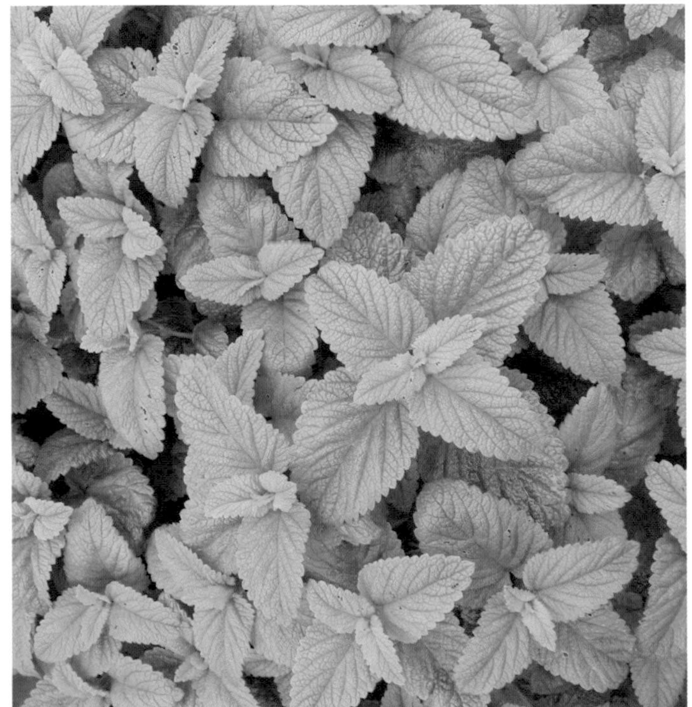

Left Melissa officinalis, or lemon balm, has calming, relaxing, sleep-promoting properties that relieve stress. Its anti-inflammatory, antivirus, antibacterial properties make it useful in treating skin virus infections including herpes.

Athlete's Foot

This is a fungal infection which mainly affects the groin and feet. Fungal infections, however, can appear anywhere on the skin, including the scalp and under the nails. It can be highly contagious and spreads easily in warm, moist places, such as bathrooms and swimming pools. To prevent the spread of infection:

- Use separate cloths and towels for each person for both washing and drying.
- Check pets for infections, as they can be a source, and treat them as necessary.
- Drink teas made from a combination of echinacea, nettles, dandelion root, burdock, and peppermint to boost immunity.
- Externally, apply oils of lavender, tea tree, or thyme. Tea tree oil can irritate the skin if used on its own so it is best used in a carrier or base oil.
- Use tinctures of myrrh, echinacea, or goldenseal on the affected area, three times a day.

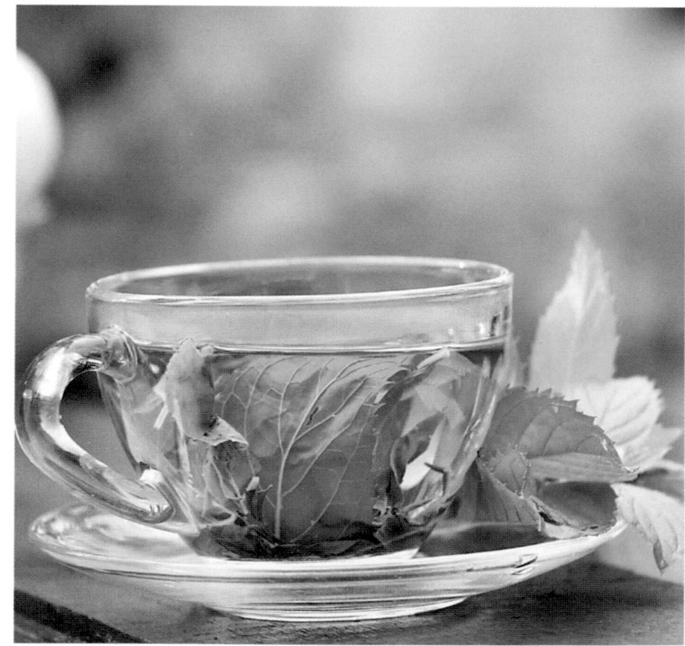

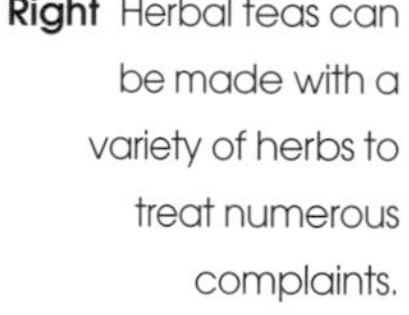

Right Herbal teas can be made with a variety of herbs to treat numerous complaints.

Chronic Fungal Infections

Fungal infections can be stubborn, and may need longterm treatment. They can appear in the form of dandruff, acne, or eczema, and professional medical diagnosis may be needed. Infections can be an indication of an imbalance in the body. Eat a healthy diet, avoiding foods that contain sugar and yeast, such as breads, cakes, alcohol, and vinegar, which encourage fungal growth. Drink pao d'arco and calendula tea instead of ordinary tea and coffee to help fight fungal infections and boost immunity. Take garlic perles and a mixture of echinacea, dandelion root, and burdock tinctures to cleanse the system. Use suggested oils and tinctures to help clear external infection.

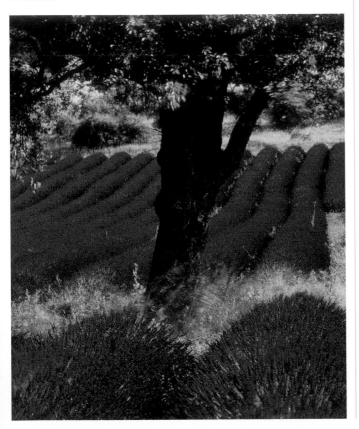

Left Lavender has many beneficial properties. Use lavender oil externally to fight fungal infections such as athlete's foot and as an antiseptic for skin infections.

Facing Page It is important to clean a cut or wound to prevent infection. A teaspoon of St. John's wort tincture in a small amount of water can be used as an antiseptic.

Wounds

Apply a cold compress to a bruise to help reduce swelling and bruising. To make a compress, soak a clean cloth in distilled witch hazel, or in 1 tsp (5 ml) of arnica or calendula tincture mixed into 8 fl oz (200 ml) water. Drink a glass of water with one drop of arnica tincture to help settle the shock. Rub arnica gel, cream, or ointment into the affected area until bruising is gone. Do not use arnica or comfrey on open wounds.

Arnica Tincture Use this tincture for the treatment of bruising and sprains. Take equal amounts of fresh arnica flowers and 70 per cent alcohol, or use one part dried flowers to 10 parts alcohol. Mix together in a glass container and seal tightly. Shake every day for two weeks, then strain the herbs through a muslin cloth. Leave this for another two days to settle, then strain again until the liquid is clear.

Burns

Immerse the burn in cold water immediately to help relieve the pain. Aloe vera is very effective in the treatment of burns as it helps to heal and cool the skin. Use it as a gel, or open the leaf of an aloe plant and rub this directly on the burn. Lavender oil or calendula ointments are also effective. Use a compress soaked in distilled witch hazel, or in an infusion of either comfrey, elderflower, or calendula, to help take away the pain and speed healing.

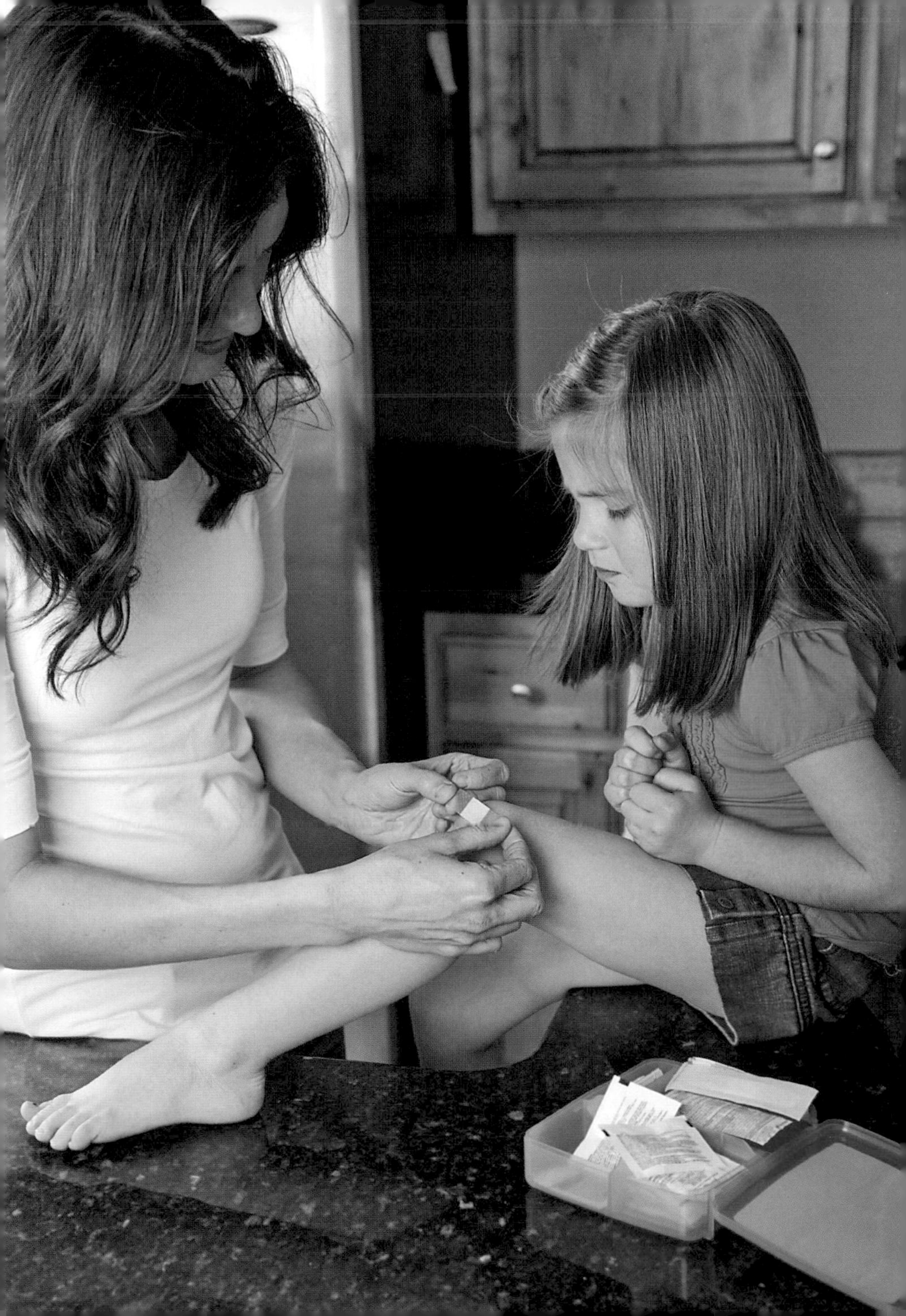

The Circulatory System

This vital system transports blood to all parts of the body. The blood carries the nutrients and oxygen that feed every cell. It then carries away the waste products, which are filtered out by the lungs, kidneys, and liver.

The heart and blood vessels make up the circulatory system. The heart acts as a pump, which takes in the oxygenated blood from the lungs and passes it out through the arteries into the finer network of vessels that feed the cells. The waste products are then returned through the blood in the veins back to the heart, where it is pumped to the lungs.

Interaction with the Body

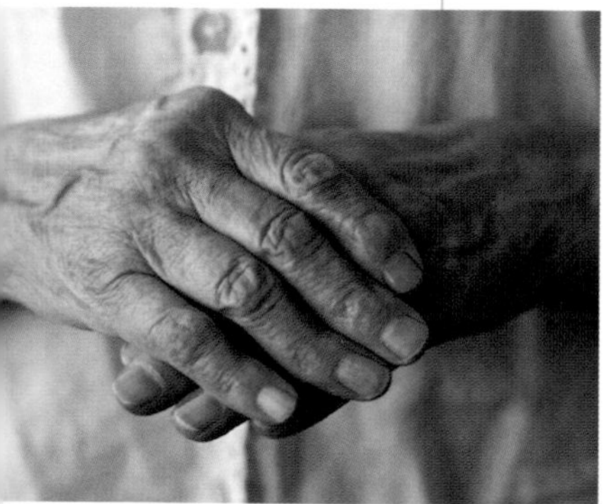

Above If the blood supply is poor then the cells in that part of the body suffer and problems and diseases very often start to occur.

Disease of any part of the body will affect the circulatory system. An organ which is damaged will cause strain on the circulation. An infection or a broken bone will need extra help to remove wastes and repair the tissue. If the circulatory system is weak, it will then cause strain on other parts of the body. Poor circulation will result in cold hands and feet, chilblains, cramps, and varicose veins. High and low blood pressure, arteriosclerosis, and palpitations put strain on the heart. These conditions can all be helped by herbal treatments and are discussed in this section.

The Chinese Medicine Approach

In traditional Chinese medicine, the heart is seen to be the "supreme controller." The heartbeat helps to steady and reassure the other parts of the body. It holds the *shen*, or spirit of peace, which guides and directs all that we do. Ailments and remedies related to a "disturbed *shen* of the heart" will be discussed in the section on the Nervous System (see pp.144–157). Chinese remedies for nourishing the blood are included here. These will be helpful in the treatment of anemia and poor circulation.

How the Circulatory System Works

The cardiovascular system is the transport system of the body, carrying respiratory gases, foodstuffs, hormones, and other material to and from the body tissues.

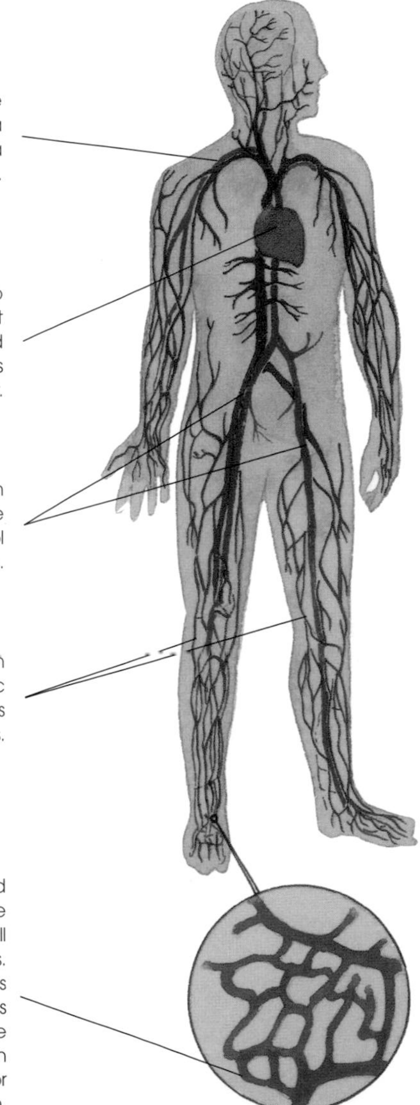

The blood is a complex fluid tissue containing specialized cells in a liquid plasma. Chinese angelica revitalizes and nourishes the blood.

The heart is a double pump containing four chambers. It pumps the blood into the blood vessels. A tea of hawthorn berries strengthens the heart.

The arteries carry blood from the heart to the tissues. Lime blossom tea clears cholesterol from the arteries.

The veins bring blood back from the tissues to the heart. Take garlic to improve circulation in cases of varicose veins.

Capillaries are minute blood vessels found throughout the tissues. They connect the small arteries to the small veins. Exchange of respiratory gases and nutrients with the tissues occurs across the walls of the capillaries. Use a foot bath with warming herbs or oils of ginger or mustard to aid poor circulation.

Prevention of Circulatory Disease

Prevention of circulatory disease is a far better option than undergoing treatment once problems have become established, and these days there is a greater emphasis on educating people about the importance of diet, exercise, and lifestyle. If we can take care of ourselves before an illness sets in, we will be happier and healthier. Herbal treatment can be used as part of a preventative program.

Low-Cholesterol Diet

Two of the most problematic foods for the circulatory system are saturated and unsaturated fat. There is strong evidence that an unhealthy, fatty diet can increase the amount of cholesterol in the blood, which may lead to arterial damage. Avoiding foods such as sugar, butter, cream, fatty meats, hard cheeses, fried foods, and eggs can help prevent a high cholesterol level. Eating a diet of fresh fruits and vegetables, wholegrains, and pulses has been shown to reduce cholesterol levels in the blood.

Smoking

Smoking is another important contributor to circulatory problems. It has a complex effect on the heart and circulation that is not fully understood. It is believed that the nicotine and carbon monoxide make the heart beat faster, while at the same time causing a thickening of the blood and an increase in the chances of its clotting. Heart attacks and poor circulation are serious problems in Western society, both related to smoking.

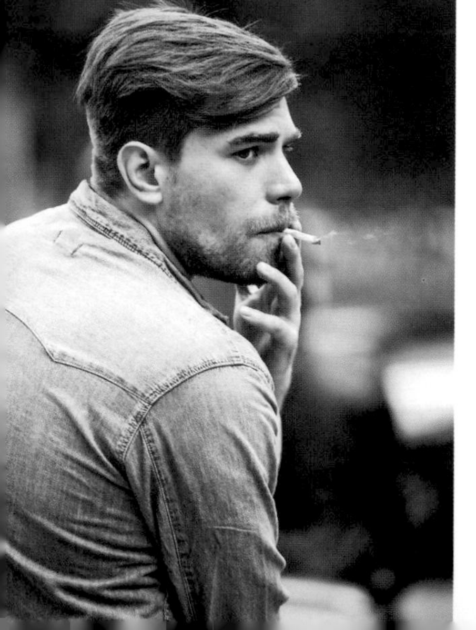

Below Smoking increases the chances of circulatory disease.

Exercise

Aerobic exercise, where the heart and lungs are put under pressure, helps to keep the circulatory system in good condition. When the heart beats faster, breathing becomes deeper and the blood is pumped into all parts of our body, enhancing its vitality and tone. Our lifestyle has become more sedentary; we walk less and drive more, and our work is less physically demanding. We need to make a conscious effort to exercise and keep fit.

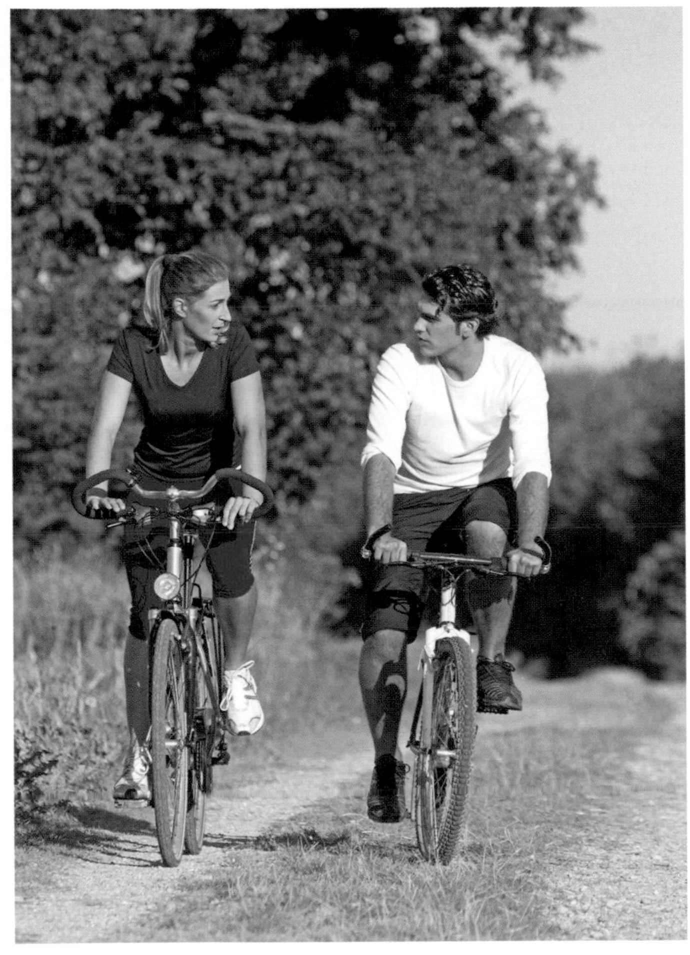

Left Physical exercise helps to keep us fit and well, especially as our lifestyle has become more sedentary.

Coping with Stress

Stress is another factor which can aggravate health problems related to the cardiovascular system. Symptoms include palpitations, chest pains and constriction, and cramping. While there are many theories on whether stress is good or bad for us, what seems to be important is how we cope with it. Herbal remedies will help to ease and alleviate symptoms of stress, but it is also necessary to understand the causes, and deal with these.

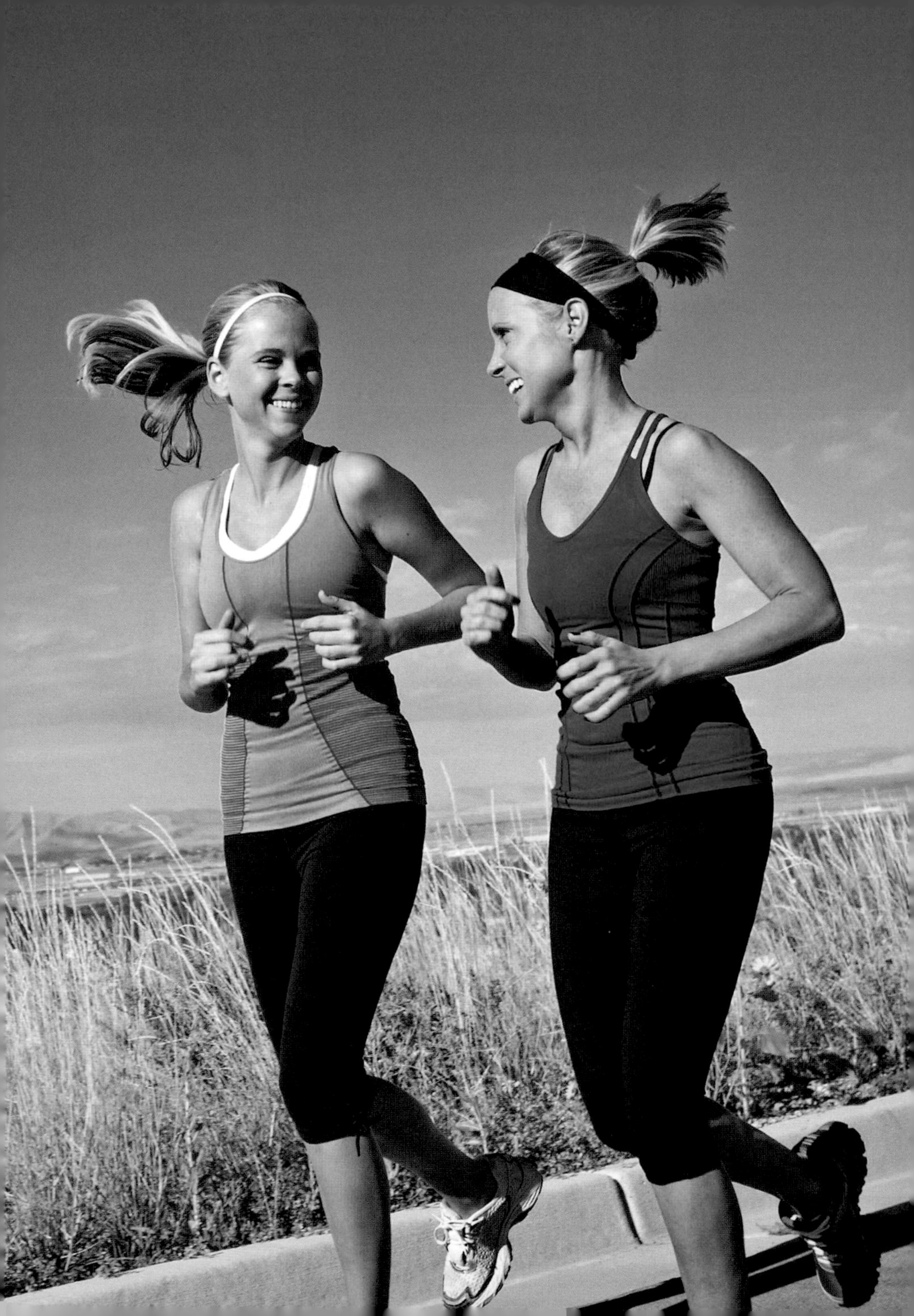

Ailments of the Circulatory System

Herbal medicine has much to offer in terms of preventing complications and easing the symptoms of circulatory problems. In this section, conditions which affect the heart, such as palpitations, arteriosclerosis, and high and low blood pressure, are discussed, as well as those which affect the periphery circulation, such as varicose veins, cold hands and feet, chilblains, and cramping. Suggestions of blood tonics for anemia are also given. More serious heart problems should always be treated under medical supervision.

Facing Page Jogging is a good way to raise your heart rate and boost your circulation.

Palpitations

A fast or irregular heartbeat may have many causes, and in most cases does not place any strain on the heart. Fear, excitement, stress, and anxiety may all cause palpitations. If they occur frequently and regularly, it is important to consult a professional medical practitioner. A diagnosis of nervous tachycardia would indicate that the palpitations are due to stress and anxiety. These can be unsettling, and herbal treatment will help to relax and steady the heartbeat. Just as important, it is necessary to give up nicotine and caffeine, because they stimulate and excite the heart. If you are already taking prescription heart medicines do not use hawthorn without advice from an herbal practitioner.

Herbal Treatment An infusion using two parts of motherwort added to one part valerian will make a relaxing and soothing tea (see Herbal Methods chapter, pp.20–47). If there are high levels of stress and anxiety, any of the relaxing herbs, such as skullcap, passionflower, camomile, or lime blossom may be helpful. Make an infusion using one or more of these herbs alone, or in a combination. Drink this three times a day, or as often as needed. If there is any weakness of the heart, arteriosclerosis, or heightened blood pressure, use hawthorn berries as well. They are an excellent heart tonic, and help to normalize the heart function.

Arteriosclerosis

This is a condition whereby the artery walls thicken and harden. Initially, deposits of calcium restrict the flow of blood to the cells. Cholesterol and fatty deposits "cling" to these deposits, which causes a degeneration of the artery walls. They can build up in the aorta, and in the arteries of the heart and brain.

Prevention Arteriosclerosis is one of the most common causes of death in the Western world. It can be aggravated by high blood pressure, a diet high in fats, lack of exercise, the excessive consumption of tea, coffee and alcohol, and also by smoking. Include foods in your diet which lower cholesterol, such as soya beans, tofu, bran, and oats, lemons, garlic, leeks and onions, and seeds.

Herbal Treatment This includes the use of lime blossom, which guards against the deposition of cholesterol with long-term use. The treatment can be taken as a tea three times a day over a period of time Hawthorn berries will strengthen the heart muscle, while yarrow or dandelion root will act as a diuretic, helping to circulate the blood through the kidneys to avoid water retention

Below To monitor blood pressure effectively, readings should be taken over a period of time.

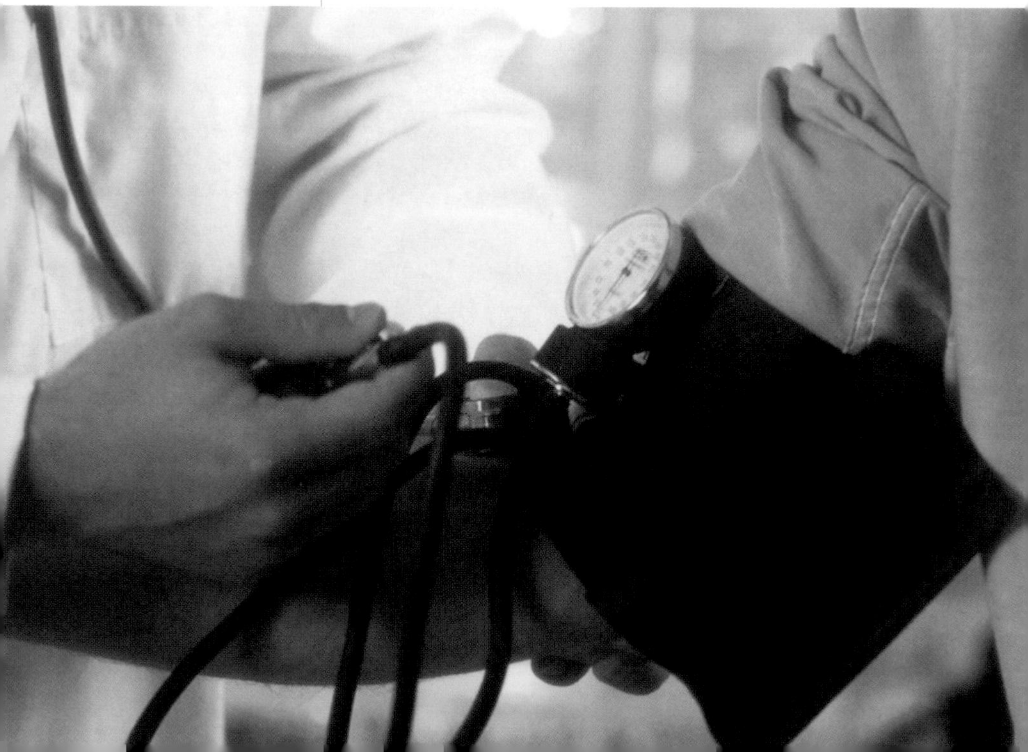

Blood Pressure

Our blood pressure fluctuates throughout the day, depending on what we are doing. Stress and anxiety may affect blood pressure. Often the process of taking the blood pressure itself will cause it to rise, especially if there is a stressful wait beforehand. It is important to monitor blood pressure over a period of time. Treatment in the early stages can be very helpful in preventing hypertension from becoming a permanent condition that needs daily medication.

Monitoring Blood Pressure

Our blood pressure fluctuates during the day depending on what we are doing. Stress and anxiety may cause blood pressure to rise and so the act of having blood pressure taken can cause a rise in blood pressure. It is important to monitor blood pressure over a period of time.

High Blood Pressure (Hypertension)

Hypertension is a common condition that needs monitoring once it becomes established. It may be caused by a wide range of physical conditions, but can also have no known cause. There are several factors that can contribute to hypertension, one being a genetic predisposition. Although this can not be altered, there are several precautions which can help to maintain healthy blood pressure.

Relaxation and Exercise Emotional problems, general stress and tension cause muscular constriction, which can tighten the blood vessels and influence the heartbeat. Relaxation, yoga, and massage can help the body to release tension and increase circulation. Herbal baths or aromatherapy oils such as lavender, rose, and lemon balm can be another way of letting go of stresses and strains. In addition, regular exercise helps the circulation and is a good way to unwind.

Dietary Factors A diet rich in fats and carbohydrates may be a factor in producing high cholesterol, which in turn may cause a buildup in the arteries. Avoid these, as well as tea, coffee, alcohol, and smoking. Use olive oil, and eat plenty of fresh fruit and vegetables, nuts and

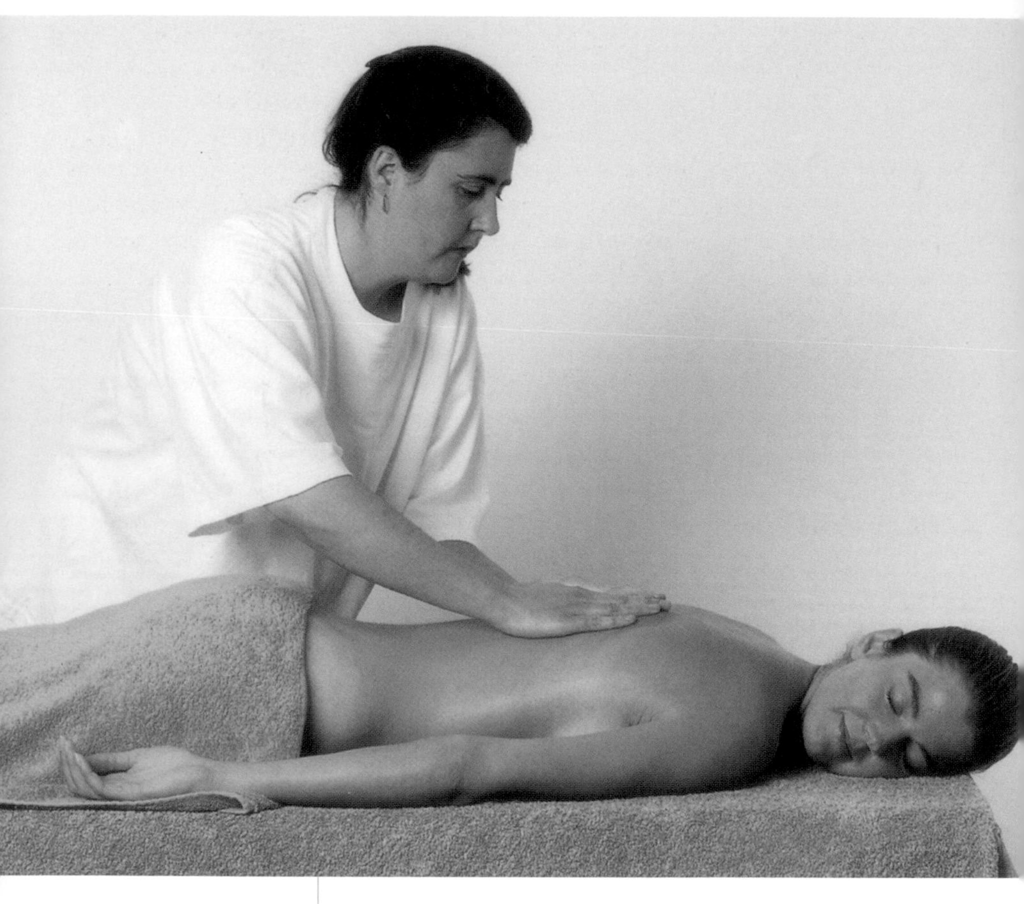

Above Massage, yoga, and other forms of relaxation can help the body to release tensions and increase circulation.

seeds, and wholegrains, as well as raw garlic or garlic perles. Over a period of time, garlic will help reduce blood pressure and lower cholesterol levels.

Herbal Treatment This includes a mixture of hawthorn berries, limeflower, nettles, and motherwort. The hawthorn berries and motherwort are tonics for the heart, and help to normalize its functions. Motherwort and limeflowers are relaxants, and limeflowers are excellent for clearing any buildup of cholesterol. Nettles are strengthening and supporting to the whole body, and help to reinvigorate the blood. Make an herbal infusion and drink 1 pint (600 ml) a day. If you are under a lot of stress, add either valerian, passionflower, or skullcap. For water retention, use diuretic herbs such as dandelion or yarrow—add them to the mixture of dried herbs. Fresh dandelion leaves can be eaten in salads.

Chinese Herbal Treatment The Chinese patent remedy *Er Ming Zuo Ci Wan,*can be used for treating hypertension. It will help to nourish the *Yin* energy, which often becomes deficient with age and overwork, and to clear symptoms of heat. These may include headache, insomnia, eye irritation, irritability, and thirst.

Low Blood Pressure (Hypotension)

This is a far less serious complaint than hypertension, however its symptoms of lethargy and tiredness can make life just as difficult. Take the herbs ginger, cayenne, or angelica as a tea or tincture (see Herbal Methods section, pp.20–47). Adding ginger and cayenne to foods can warm and stimulate the circulation. In addition, drink a tea of hawthorn berries and nettles over several weeks. These will help to regulate the blood pressure and strengthen the system. Use warming oils or herbs, such as rosemary, ginger, or cinnamon in hand and foot baths (see Herbal Methods section, pp.20–47).

Varicose Veins

The enlargement and aching of veins can be caused by too much standing, too little exercise, and the condition is often inherited. Pregnancy, constipation, and being overweight can aggravate the condition. Make sure that the feet are elevated when sitting for long periods of time to counteract the effects of gravity, and take exercise, as muscular movement helps the blood return to the heart through the veins.

Herbal Treatment Herbal medicine can help this condition when supported by exercise. A mixture of yarrow, St. John's wort, lime flower, and hawthorn berries will help to improve circulation and strengthen the veins. To ease any local inflammation, use a compress.

soaked in witch hazel, or in teas of comfrey or calendula (see Herbal Methods section, pp.20–47). For severe aching, spray the area with cold water or apply crushed ice for several seconds. Massage the muscles around this area with oils of lavender, juniper, or rosemary. Take garlic to improve circulation as well as supplements of vitamins B complex, C, E, and zinc.

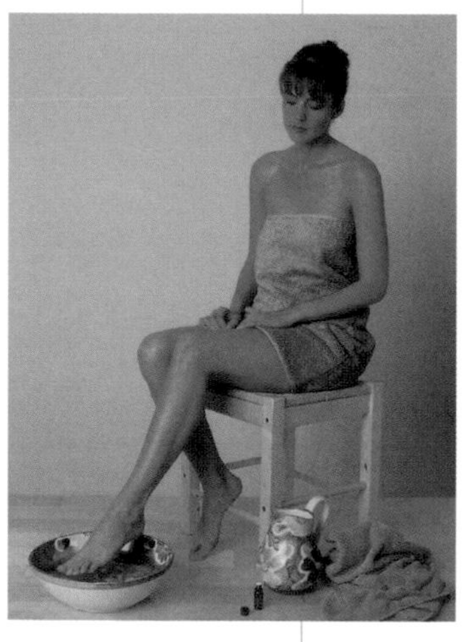

Above Foot baths are a relaxing way to help improve circulation. Add warming oils or herbs such as cinnamon, mustard, or black pepper to warm cold feet.

Poor Circulation

This can result in cold hands and feet. Exercise and eating green, leafy vegetables can help to strengthen the circulation. Use warming spices such as cinnamon, ginger, cloves, chilli, and cayenne in cooking. Add several slices of ginger root to your favorite tea. Make an infusion using equal parts of prickly ash bark or berries and hawthorn berries, and add a slice of ginger. Drink this three times a day, especially in cold weather. The prickly ash will help to stimulate the circulation, the hawthorn acts as a tonic for the circulation, and the ginger is warming. Garlic is also warming and helps to cleanse and strengthen the blood vessels.

Hand-and-Foot Baths Make a hand-and-foot bath using warming herbs or oils such as ginger, cinnamon, mustard, or black pepper (see Herbal Methods chapter, pp.20–47).

Chilblains

These are red swellings, usually found on the fingers and toes, caused by exposure to the cold. It is important to protect the hands and feet by wearing warm gloves and socks. Use rubber gloves to protect the hands if you are washing dishes, or if immersing them in cold water. If the chilblains itch, soothe them with calendula ointment or oil of lavender. If the skin is not broken, put arnica ointment, neat lemon juice, or cayenne ointment on the chilblains.

Chinese Herbal Treatment There is an excellent Chinese herbal formula for warming the extremities. It is useful in chronic conditions in which the hands and feet are cold to the touch and feel very cold to the person. It can also be helpful in the treatment of Raynaud's disease and cold rheumatic and arthritic conditions. *Dang Gui Si Ni Tang* (*Dang Gui* Decoction For Frigid Extremities) warms the channels, disperses the cold, nourishes the blood, and unblocks the blood vessels. It should be used with caution during spring and summer, in warm climates, and if there are symptoms of heat, such as a red face, hot flashes, or sensations of warmth.

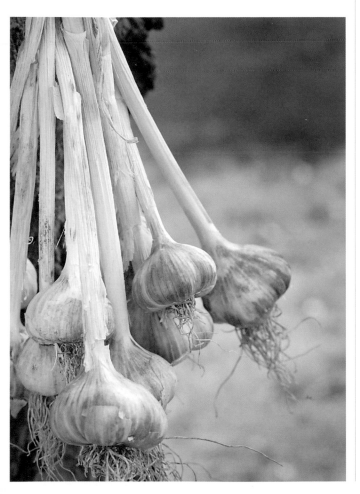

Left Garlic inhibits platelet aggregation, which can result in improved blood flow throughout the body. Other possible benefits include modest reductions in blood pressure and cholesterol levels.

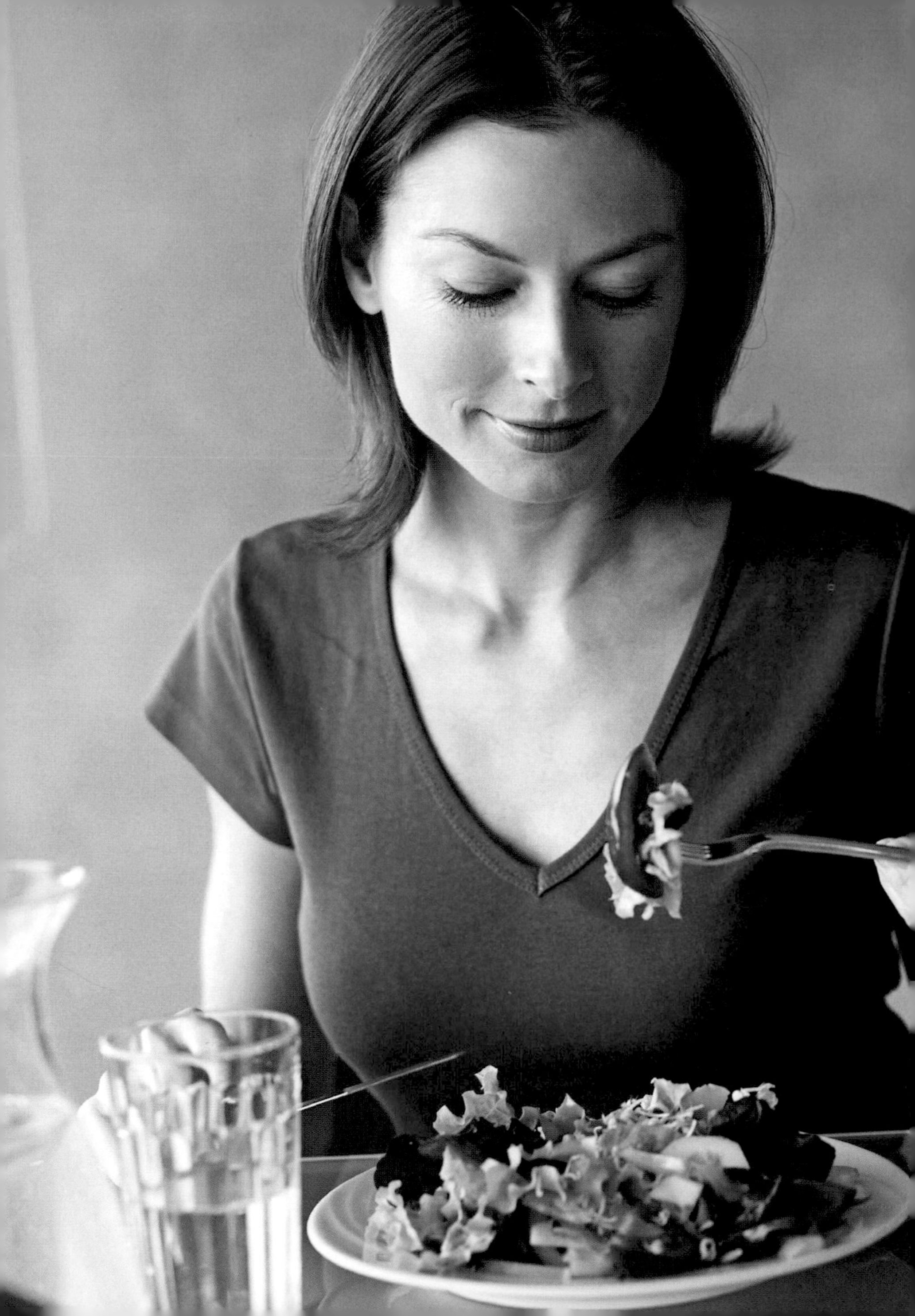

Anemia

In anemia there is a lack of oxygen-carrying hemoglobin in the blood. Anemia can be caused by a loss of blood, an inherited abnormality of the red blood cells, or an inability to produce red blood cells. Symptoms include: tiredness, dizziness, shortness of breath, paleness, and headaches. The four main types of anemia are iron deficiency, pernicious, megaloblastic, and sickle-cell. A simple blood test will reveal if anemia is present. It is then important to find its cause, for which professional medical attention is needed.

Types of Anemia Anemia caused by an iron deficiency is the most common form. This can be the result of poor diet, loss of blood, illness, and infection. Pernicious anemia is due to a lack of vitamin B12. Megaloblastic anemia occurs because of a shortage of folic acid, one of the many B vitamins. Sickle-cell anemia is an inherited blood disorder most commonly found in people of Afro-Caribbean and Middle Eastern origin; this needs professional medical treatment.

Dietary Factors Dietary and herbal treatments can help revitalize the blood. Eating plenty of iron-rich foods such as dark-green, leafy vegetables, walnuts, raisins, parsley, apricots, and pumpkin seeds, and drinking red wine in moderation, will all help.

Herbal Treatment Herbal teas of chickweed, nettle, and dandelion leaves, and decoctions of burdock and yellow dock root will all replenish the blood. Drink three cups a day using one or several of the herbs in combination (see Herbal Methods chapter, pp.20–47).

Medicinal Wine The treatment of anemia can be helped with a medicinal wine of 8 oz (200 g) yellow dock, 2 tsp (4 g) of licorice root, 2 tsp (4 g) of juniper berries, 2 oz (50 g) dried nettles, 2 oz (50 g) chopped dried apricots, and 4 oz (100 g) of sugar added to 2 pints (1 liter) of red wine. Allow to soak for two weeks, then strain and put into a sterilized bottle. Drink one sherry glassful a day on an empty stomach. (See also medicinal wines in the Herbal Methods chapter, pp.20–47.)

Facing page Making sure your diet is healthy can go a long way toward circulatory health.

The Musculoskeletal System

The bones and muscles give shape and form to the body. Their movement and strength vary with each individual and with age, determining physical ability throughout life. It is important to maintain the good health of the bones and muscles, especially as we grow older.

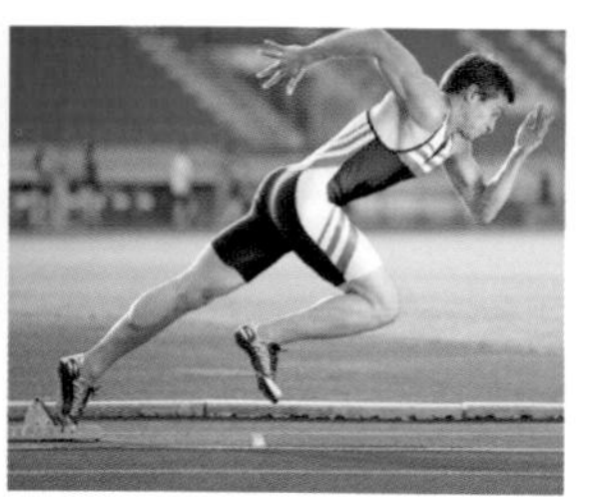

Above Muscular activity accounts for much of the body's energy consumption so for athletes it is particularly important to support muscle repair and growth.

The adult skeleton consists of 206 bones, made of living tissue that is rich in blood and nerves. Bones are living things that grow and repair themselves. Muscles account for half an adult's body weight; their primary function is to allow the skeleton to move. Muscles may be attached directly to the bones, or connected by tendons. The muscles and tendons act as part of a muscle group controlled by the nervous system.

Interaction with the Body

Muscles and bones form a framework that protects and holds the vital organs of the body in place. The bones are a reservoir of calcium, phosphorous, sodium, and other elements. Red and white blood cells are produced within bone marrow. The bones, muscles, and tendons maintain their strength and suppleness through exercise and nutrients from our diet. Many of the chronic ailments affecting this system are related to these two factors.

The Chinese Medicine Approach

In traditional Chinese medicine there are several energies that relate to the muscles and bones. The bones are connected with the kidney *qi*, or energy; the muscles to the spleen *qi*; the tendons to the liver and gallbladder *qi*. Ailments related to muscles, bones, and tendons may involve treatments for these different energies, but may also include herbs to nourish the blood and aid circulation. Such ailments are described as being "hot" or "cold," and cooling or warming herbs will be part of the treatment, respectively. For example, stiff, cold arthritic joints will require the use of warming and strengthening herbs; red, swollen, hot joints will need herbs that clear heat and toxicity.

How the Musculoskeletal System Works

The skeleton provides a rigid framework to support the body and maintain its shape. The main function of the skeleton is to provide a system of levers, moved by skeletal muscle, allowing the body to move. Skeletal muscle makes up about half the weight of the average adult. The skeletal muscles are, with a few exceptions, attached to the bone, either directly or via tendons. They move the bones at their joints when they contract. The muscles only exert power during contraction. Several muscles are attached around a joint to permit a variety of opposing movements.

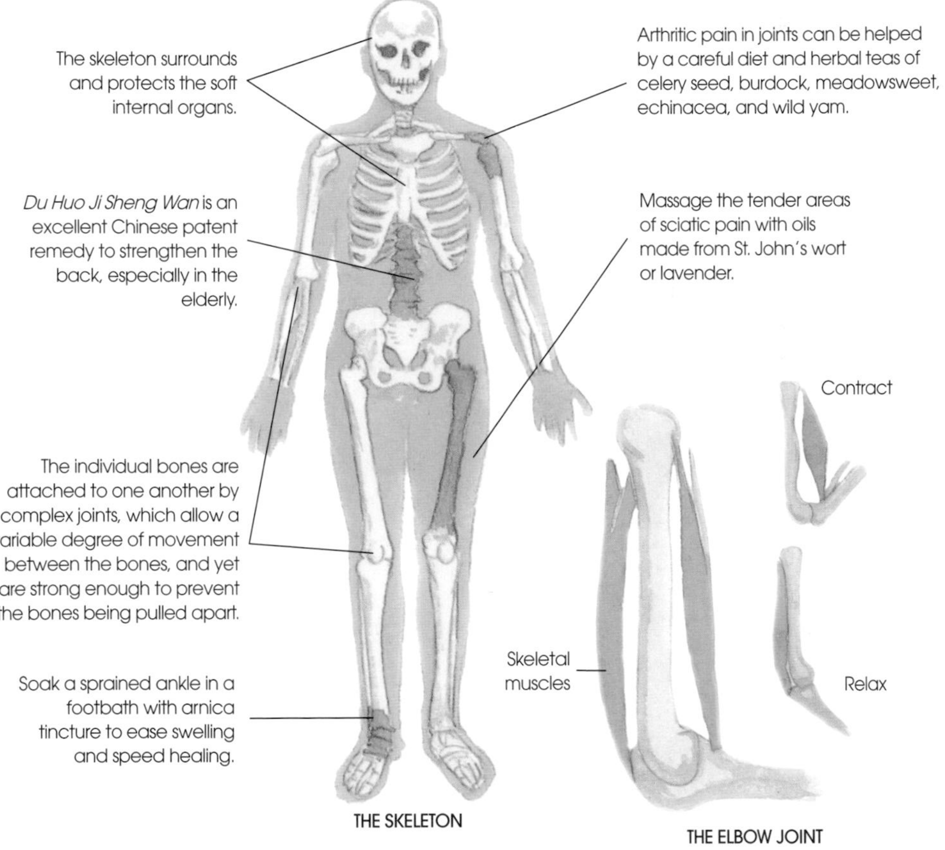

The skeleton surrounds and protects the soft internal organs.
Du Huo Ji Sheng Wan is an excellent Chinese patent remedy to strengthen the back, especially in the elderly.
The individual bones are attached to one another by complex joints, which allow a variable degree of movement between the bones, and yet are strong enough to prevent the bones being pulled apart.
Soak a sprained ankle in a footbath with arnica tincture to ease swelling and speed healing.
Arthritic pain in joints can be helped by a careful diet and herbal teas of celery seed, burdock, meadowsweet, echinacea, and wild yam.
Massage the tender areas of sciatic pain with oils made from St. John's wort or lavender.
Contract
Relax
Skeletal muscles

THE SKELETON

THE ELBOW JOINT

Prevention of Disorders

The health of the musculoskeletal system is affected by the way we use it. Good posture, exercise, and a healthy diet all contribute to long-term health. The Alexander Technique and yoga can help to promote healthy posture and keep the muscles and joints supple. A great deal can be done to heal structural problems with the use of osteopathy or chiropractics, especially those resulting from accidents or injuries. Emotional stress and tension can cause rigidity of the bones and muscles; these should be dealt with before they bring about a serious condition.

Ailments of the Musculoskeletal System

Rheumatism, arthritis, and gout are conditions commonly found in the elderly. Herbal treatments and diet will be suggested for these ailments. Treatments for backache and sciatica will be given, with some herbs to be taken as teas, and others to be used in a soothing herbal bath. Cramps and sprains are usually temporary conditions, and suggestions will be given to ease discomfort.

Rheumatism and Arthritis

Both of these conditions have symptoms of painful, swollen, and stiff joints. Often the conditions are inherited, and symptoms occur as a result of the body's inability to cope with an inappropriate diet and a stressful life. Rheumatism and arthritis can be the result of an injury or accident. Constant strain from physical work may cause an arthritic condition later on, such as the arthritic shoulder of a builder who has carried bricks on his back for many years. The weather often plays a role, with the cold and damp having the most negative impact.

Dietary Factors One of the causes of rheumatism and arthritis is an accumulation of toxins and waste products in the joints, which an inappropriate diet can aggravate. Generally, foods that cause an acidic reaction in the stomach should be avoided: red meats, eggs and dairy products, vinegar, refined sugar, and many spices. Foods high in oxalic acid, such as rhubarb, gooseberries, and black and red currants, should also not be eaten. In some cases, food allergies can result in arthritis and an elimination diet may help. This is best done with advice from a professional dietician. Herbal teas should be substituted for coffee, tea, and alcohol. Include fresh fruit and vegetables, and drink 3 pints (1½ liters) of water daily. Add a teaspoon of cider vinegar to a glass of water and drink this every morning.

Herbal Treatment A tea made from a combination of celery seed, burdock, meadowsweet, and echinacea will help to clear waste. Add wild yam or devil's claw to reduce pain and swelling. If there is constipation, drink aloe vera juice, or take a decoction of yellow dock and licorice (see Herbal Methods chapter, pp.20–47). Take supplements of evening primrose oil or cod liver oil to keep joints supple. Rub joints with oils of lavender, rosemary, peppermint, and arnica.

Chinese Herbal Treatment A sweet-tasting traditional Chinese herbal remedy that is useful for easing stiffness, especially in the elderly, can be made from lycium fruit (*gou qi zi*) and Chinese licorice (*gan cao*). Combine 1 oz (20 g) lycium fruit with ½ oz (10 g) licorice in a pot with 1½ pints (750 ml) water. Simmer gently for 30 minutes, then strain. Drink half in the morning and the other half in the evening. The lycium fruit will nourish the blood, while the licorice will strengthen the *qi*, or energy.

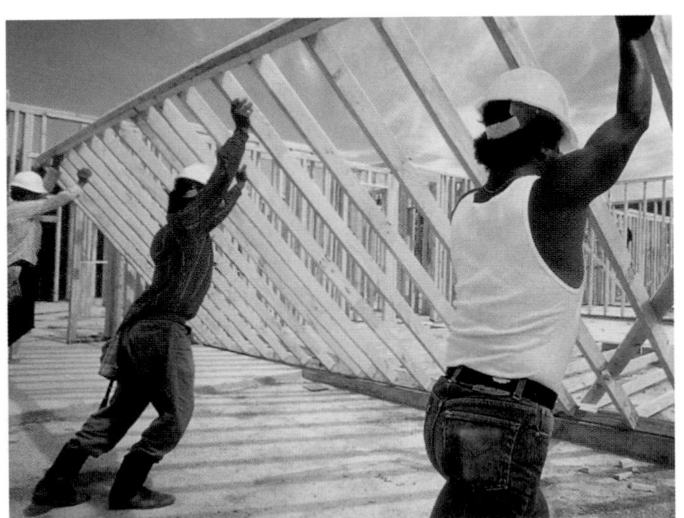

Below Rheumatism and arthritis may develop in later years from strain on one part of the body, or as a result of an injury.

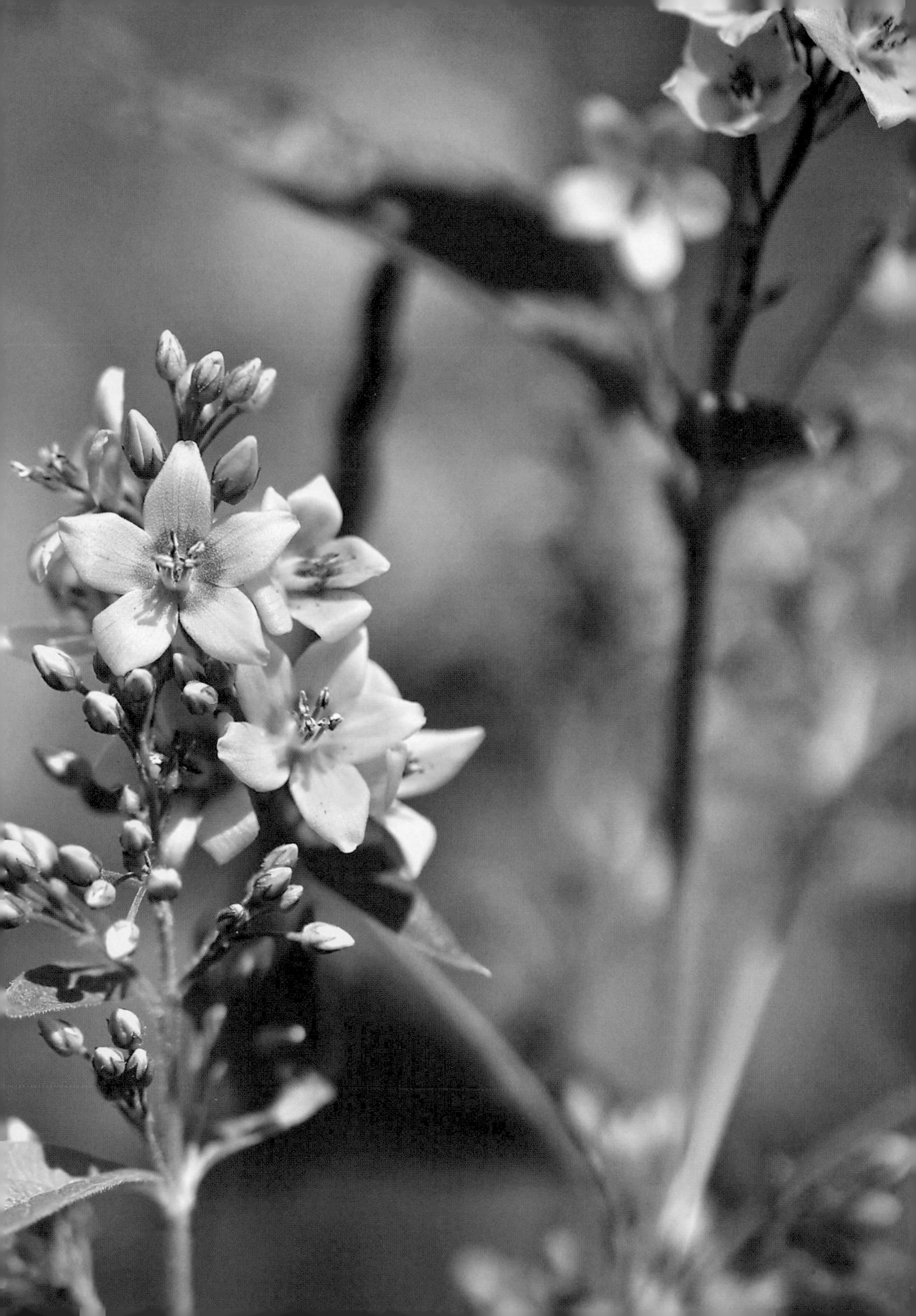

Gout

This is a specific joint problem caused by a buildup of uric acid in the body. It can be a very painful condition, which often affects the feet. Herbal treatment includes a combination of anti-rheumatic herbs and diuretics to aid the process of elimination via the kidneys. Use equal amounts of burdock root, celery seed, and yarrow to make a decoction. Drink it three times a day over a period of time (see Herbal Methods section, pp.20–47).

Dietary Factors Diet is of primary importance in the treatment of gout. Avoid any foods that encourage the body's production of uric acid, such as sardines, anchovies, crab and shellfish, as well as liver, kidneys, and beans. Coffee and tea, and especially alcohol, should not be drunk. Gout may be helped by taking folic acid and vitamin C supplements.

Backache

This can have many causes, and it should be investigated to help determine the best treatment. If it is the result of strained muscles caused by a sudden, violent movement or overuse, massage the area with oils of lavender, rosemary, or St. John's wort to help relieve stiffness and pain. A hot bath with a strong herbal infusion of camomile will help the muscles to relax. Use hot compresses soaked in crampbark, valerian, or ginger frequently. Make a hot salt compress by heating salt in a frying pan and wrapping it in a soft cloth. The salt will hold the heat, which will help to relax muscle spasm.

ChineseHerbal Treatment *Du Huo Ji Sheng Wan* is a patent remedy that is good for treating chronic backache, sciatica, arthritis, and rheumatism. It contains herbs to strengthen the body, and is often used for older people. It should not be used with hot, swollen joints, fevers, or night sweats. It is helpful for ailments that are made worse by the cold and damp. Another Chinese herbal remedy for weakness and pain in the lower back is *Liu Wei Di Huang Wan*. It is used for conditions such as restlessness, insomnia, mild night sweats, dizziness, tinnitus, high blood pressure, and burning in the soles and palms.

Facing page
St John's wort is used as a topical remedy for wounds, abrasions, burns, and muscle pain, the hyperforin has both antibacterial and anti-inflammatory properties.

Right Lavender or St. John's wort oil can help to ease back or neck pain, but professional help from a chiropractor or osteopath may be needed.

Sciatica

This is an inflammation of the sciatic nerve, which runs from the buttock down the back of the leg into the calf. Sciatica can cause intense pain and tenderness. It is often due to a problem in the lower back, and osteopathic or chiropractic treatment may be essential. Some cases of sciatica are caused by neuralgia, or nerve pain, and treatment using nerve relaxants and tonics may be helpful. Drink teas of camomile, passionflower, and valerian to help soothe the inflammation and relax the muscles surrounding the nerve. Add skullcap and vervain to support the nervous system. Massage the buttock and leg with lavender and St. John's wort oil to relieve the pain (see Herbal Methods section, pp.20–47, for nerve tonic oil recipe, and below, right, for treatment using *moxa*.)

Sprains

Muscles, ligaments, and tendons can be pulled as a result of injury, causing a sprain. Soak in a hot bath with rosemary or thyme to increase circulation to the injured area. Arnica tincture can be used to make a hot compress or bath. Use 1 tsp (5 ml) in 1 pint (600 ml) water (see Herbal Methods section, pp.20–47). Soak the sprain for 15 minutes in the solution, repeating every four hours. Arnica gel, cream, or ointment will also help, but do not use if the skin is broken.

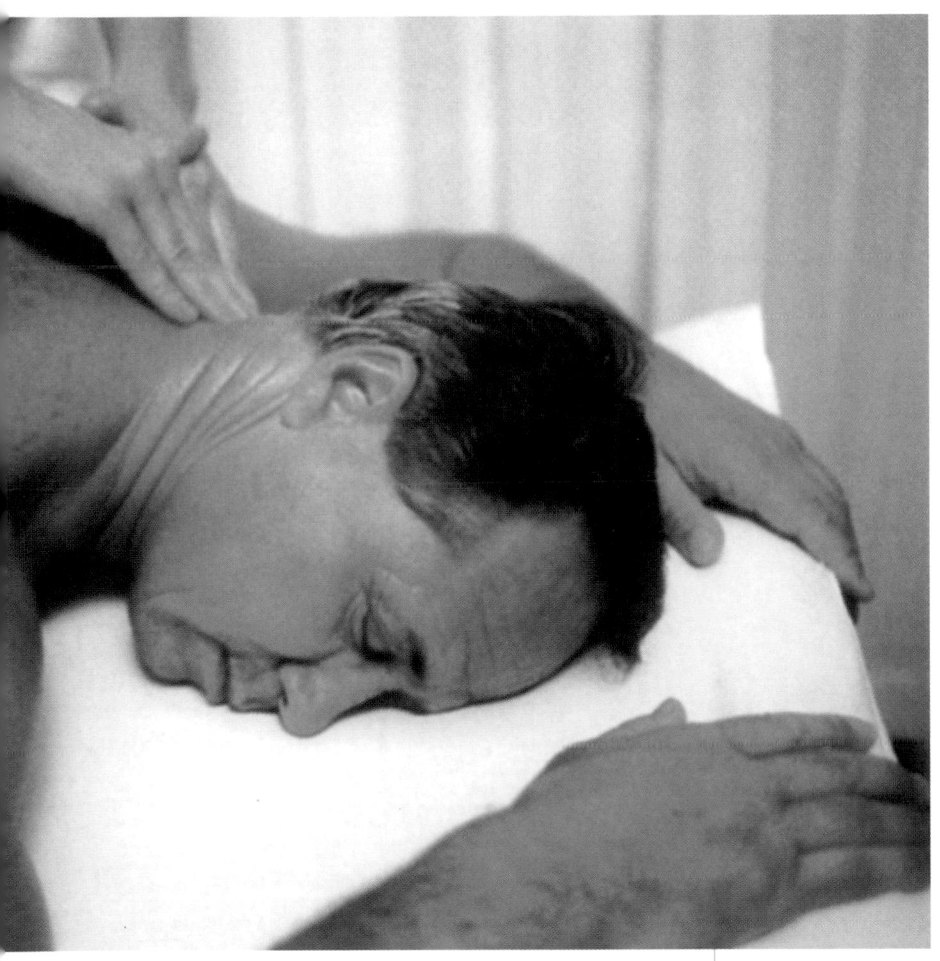

Mugwort (*Moxa*) This can be obtained in stick form, which is called a "*moxa* roll". The dried herb is compressed and rolled in paper to make an herbal "cigar." When lit, the "cigar" is placed near the painful area, which is warmed for 10 minutes, twice a day. (To extinguish the *moxa* roll, cut off the lit end and let it drop into a bowl of water.) *Moxa* can also be used to relieve back pain and sciatica. Use acupuncture with the *moxa* in order to speed up relief.

The Nervous System

A holistic approach is one that recognizes the interaction of the physical and psychological, with the nervous system as the link. Symptoms of stress may have a physical reaction, but it is the nervous system that helps us to cope with stress.

The nervous system helps the body to communicate and control its different parts. It is made up of the brain, the nerve cells, and the nerve fibers. It coordinates our physical reactions, controls the involuntary muscles and organs such as those used in breathing, and helps us to interpret and react to our environment through the senses.

The Emotional Aspect

In today's society there are many demands and pressures made on us, involving work and family commitments. It is the nervous system which takes the strain and helps us to cope with a way of life that is becoming ever faster and more complicated. Every aspect of our lives, from what we eat to where we live, involves greater choices and more difficult decisions than even a generation ago. Taking care of ourselves means making a conscious effort to relax and enjoy our lives. This is sometimes very difficult to do in a society where neuroses can seem to be the only possible reaction to its demands. Herbal treatment can be one way of helping to achieve some emotional stability in a fast-changing world.

Below Taking time to relax and enjoy life eases the stress and tension that can have a negative effect on the nervous system.

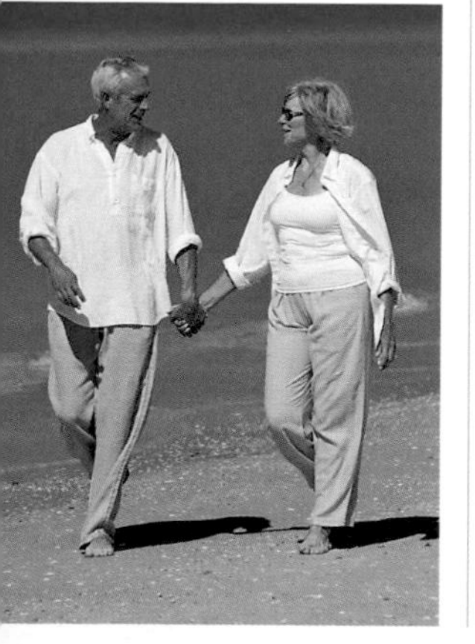

Affecting the Body

There are a number of physical ailments that have a strong relationship to the nervous system. These include high blood pressure, coronary disease, asthma, indigestion, ulcers, skin rashes, and menstrual problems. In treating these ailments, it is useful to include herbs that relax and support the nervous system. These are discussed in other sections of the book, but it may be useful to consider some of the herbs suggested here, especially if stress and anxiety make these conditions worse.

How the Nervous System Works

The nervous system consists of the brain, nerve cells, and nerve fibers. It conducts messages to and from the brain and around the body, and also helps maintain homeostasis, or balance, within the body.

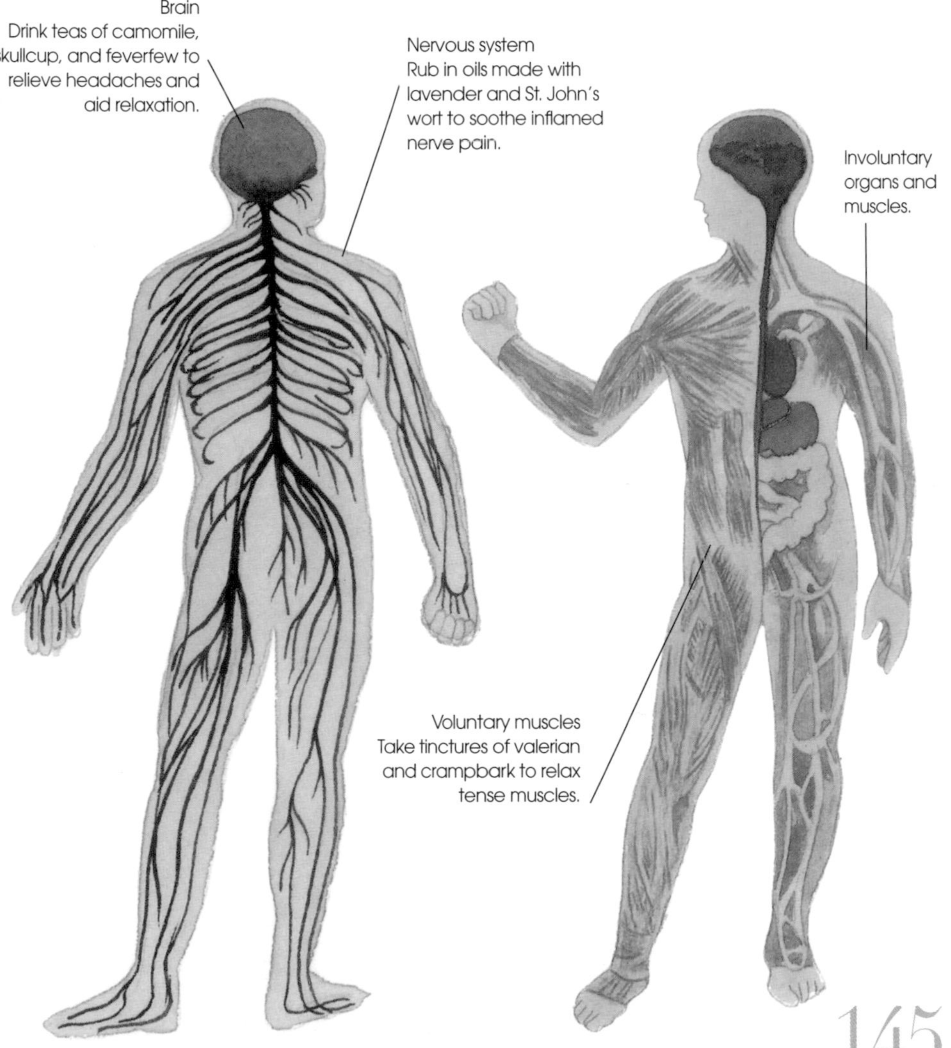

Brain
Drink teas of camomile, skullcup, and feverfew to relieve headaches and aid relaxation.
Nervous system
Rub in oils made with lavender and St. John's wort to soothe inflamed nerve pain.
Involuntary organs and muscles.
Voluntary muscles
Take tinctures of valerian and crampbark to relax tense muscles.

The Chinese Medicine Approach

In traditional Chinese medicine, disorders of the nervous system are seen as the result of disturbances of *shen*, or the spirit of the heart. The heart is considered to be the "supreme controller," and a calm, steady heartbeat tells the body that all is well. Stress and anxiety, insomnia, or hyperactivity can affect the heartbeat and disturb the *shen* of the heart. According to traditional Chinese medicine, these types of disorders can also come from a deficiency or stagnation of *qi*, or energy. For example, depression can be the result of tiredness,

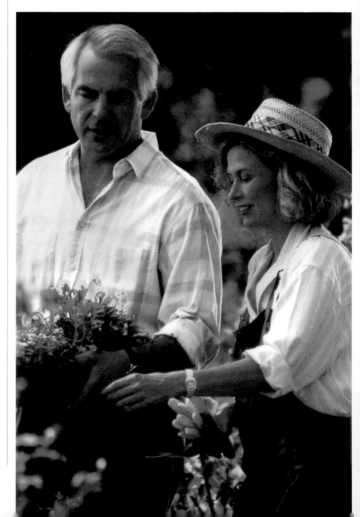

Right Gardening, walking, and sports are all enjoyable ways to relax, exercise, breathe fresh air, and, at the same time, relieve tensions.

or may be caused by lethargy or inactivity. Many times it comes from an interaction between the two.

Relaxation

Relaxation and meditation are two ways of relieving stress and tension. When a state of peace is felt in the body and the mind, healing can take place. Even if this is just for one hour a day, it can have a profound effect on the rest of daily life. There are many ways of relaxing, including gardening, listening to music, or taking a walk. What is important is to take time to forget about worries and cares.

Bodywork

Exercise is another important way of helping to support the nervous system. Tense muscles restrict blood flow and breathing. Whether it is a vigorous game of squash or a gentle hour of yoga, the muscles will relax and feelings of well-being will return. Massage, aromatherapy, and other therapies that work on the body help to keep us supple and our bodies at ease.

Counseling

Psychotherapy and counseling can help to increase our understanding of our responses to difficult situations. Past traumas and negative patterns can hinder our ability to sort out problems in a positive way. Talking with others can give us new ideas for coping with stressful events. It is important to feel that others care and listen to us, especially in a society in which other people are becoming increasingly anonymous.

Caffeine and Nicotine

These are both stimulants. They cause the heart to beat faster and the adrenal glands to produce more adrenaline. In a crisis the body does this naturally, so there is enough energy to cope. Coffee, tea, and smoking nicotine place a strain on the body by continually creating this effect. In the long run, this can lead to tiredness and ill health; it is the body's way of saying "stop." Herbal teas can be a delicious and healthy substitute to caffeine drinks, and a way to replenish our energy.

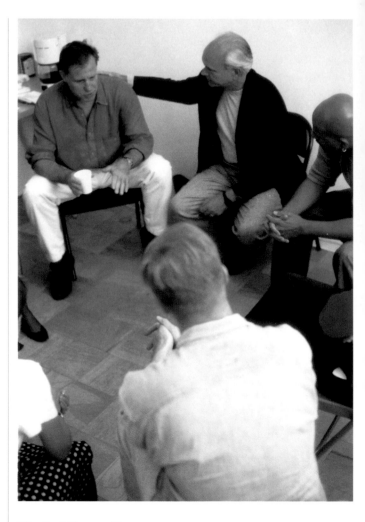

Right Talking with others who can identify with your problems may help to bring new solutions to traumatic and stressful situations.

Herbal Remedies

These are very effective in helping to support the nervous system through the use of nervine tonics, such as ginseng, skullcap, oats, and vervain. Nervine relaxants include camomile, crampbark, hops, hyssop, lavender, lime blossom, motherwort, passionflower, St. John's wort, skullcap, and valerian. Some of these help to relax the muscles and soothe the nerves to create a feeling of ease.

Ailments of the Nervous System

Herbal treatments for each of the following disorders are discussed below: stress and anxiety, depression, insomnia, hyperactivity, headache and migraine, neuralgia, and nervous exhaustion.

Stress

This is the body's natural reaction to any situation that places extra demands on us. It can have a positive or negative effect, depending on our response. Long-term stress, however, can put strain on the nervous system and other areas of the body that may be weak or prone to reacting to stress. Herbs can help to prevent debility and give you the energy needed to make positive choices in stressful situations. Nerve tonics, such as skullcap and vervain, can be taken as teas and help to strengthen the nervous system. Oats, taken daily as porridge or gruel, are an essential part of the treatment, especially if there is general debility. Vitamins C and B-complex are also useful during stressful times.

Ginseng This is another important nerve tonic that is used when there are other symptoms of weakness. It is classified as an adaptogen. These help improve the body's ability to adapt to different situations, enabling it to avoid reaching a breaking point or collapse. Take it as a Chinese decoction, tincture, medicinal wine, or powder in capsules.

Anxiety

This condition can be the result of ongoing stress or a traumatic event in our lives. Sometimes it can become a habitual response, even to situations where there is no cause for worry. Using herbs to help ease feelings of anxiety reminds us of the strength that comes from feeling peaceful in our daily lives. An herbal decoction of valerian, skullcap, and verbena calms anxiety and builds up the nervous system. Herbal baths in lavender, rosemary, or camomile help to ease tensions. Drink infusions of lime blossom, camomile, passionflower, hops, hyssop, or motherwort to replace caffeine drinks such as coffee and black tea.

Right Herbal teas are a good way to take a range of herbs that can help relieve tensions and mood depressions.

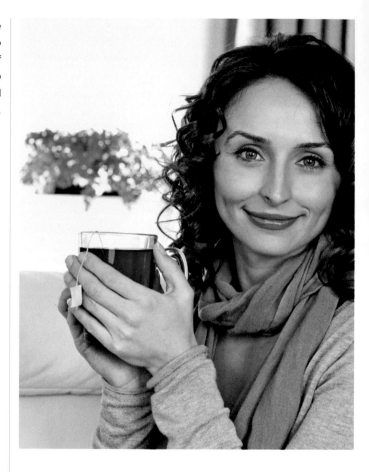

Depression

This can be the result of a long-term physical illness, general tiredness, or difficulties caused by external forces. Herbal treatment can help to lift the depression and strengthen the body, creating a more positive attitude to cope with its other causes. If there is general debility with the depression, try a Chinese herbal decoction of ginseng (see p.42). Take wild oats, skullcap, or vervain daily as teas or tinctures to help lift the spirits and replace nutrients. For depression following an illness, drink a tea made from rosemary, vervain, and dandelion leaves. Gingko is another herbal supplement that helps to alleviate depression, especially in the elderly. Since depression can be a serious problem, professional treatment using commercially prepared, standardized extracts may be necessary. In this case, be sure to consult a health professional.

Seasonal Affective Disorder (SAD)
St. John's wort will help to brighten moods and has recently been used to treat SAD, in which depression sets in during the winter months. Add this to other herbs used for treating depression to make a medicinal tea or tincture.

Insomnia
Sleepless nights can be caused by tension, anxiety, overwork, physical pain, too much caffeine, and too little fresh air and exercise. Insomnia can create all sorts of other problems, such as chronic tiredness, lack of concentration, and depression. A good night's rest is healing for both the body and the mind.

Herbal Treatment A warm herbal bath before bed, using lavender, lime flower, camomile, or rose will ease tense muscles and calm an overactive mind. Try drinking camomile as a tea or tincture before bed (see Herbal Methods section, pp.20–47). Other herbs that can be taken as infusions are lime blossom, catnip, lemon balm, or hops. Sleep pillows of lavender, rose petals, or hops can be tucked under your pillow at night. For persistent insomnia, try a combination of passionflower, valerian, and hops as a tincture. Take half a teaspoon in a small amount of water one hour before bedtime and repeat if you wake.

Chinese Herbal Treatment Chinese herbal patent formulae have several remedies that are useful for insomnia. *Suan Zao Ren Tang Pian* helps to treat insomnia with mental agitation, restlessness, and irritability. It calms the *shen*, the spirit of the heart. *Tian Wang Bu Xin Wan* (Heavenly King Benefit Heart Pill) also calms the *shen* and helps with insomnia that may come after a long illness or with aging. It can be used to treat insomnia and other symptoms due to a hyperactive thyroid.

Hyperactivity

This is a growing concern among parents of young children. Lack of concentration, an inability to sit still, temper tantrums, and sleep difficulties can all be symptoms. It varies with each child, but it often has a traumatic effect on both the child and the parent. A combination of good diet and herbal treatment aids this problem.

Dietary Factors Provide a diet that is as pure and natural as possible, avoiding artificial colorings and additives, which are now required by law to be listed on packaged foods. Notice if any foods spark off reactions in the child, since hyperactivity can be related to food allergies. Make sure that he or she has plenty of fresh air and exercise to help them let off steam.

Herbal Treatment An herbal tea of red clover should be drunk three times a day over a period of time to eliminate any toxicity from the body. Red clover is also a nervine relaxant. If stronger relaxants are needed, use oats and vervain as well. Oats can be given as porridge and the vervain as a tea or tincture. Relaxing herbal baths, using camomile or lavender, help to calm the child before bed. Try a vaporizer or aromatherapy oil burner with these herbs or essential oils to create a peaceful atmosphere at bedtime (see Herbal Methods chapter, pp.20–47).

Relieving Stress, Tension and Anxiety

There are four main ways of helping to relieve the symptoms of stress. It depends how serious the problem is and on the personality of the sufferer as to what the most effective cure might be. Sometimes a combination of two or more of the approaches might be an effective way to help. If you feel that self-help methods are not for you, or that your problem is too severe, your first port of call should be your own doctor, who will then be able to refer you on to other specialists, should this be necessary.

If your symptoms are fairly mild—perhaps you feel a bit down or stressed due to work pressures—then you might try some of the body work suggestions. For example, yoga, when practised daily can soon show remarkable de-stressing results, and the Alexander technique can affect well-being subtly through adjustments to posture and body-carriage. Spiritual healing, such as meditation or prayer, can be effective over a long period and so may be useful for helping long-term feelings of tension in one's attitude to life in general. However, if your problems seem more serious, medicinal help and possibly psychotherapy may be the best course of action.

Psychotherapeutic Approaches:
- Counseling
- Hypnotherapy
- Psychiatry
- Tender loving care (TLC)

Medicinal Approaches:
- Herbal medicine
- Homeopathy
- Diet
- Bach Flower Remedies

Spiritual Approaches
- Prayer
- Meditation
- Music
- Poetry
- Gardening
- Country walks
- Tranquility

Working on the body:
- Exercise
- Massage
- Yoga
- Herbal baths
- Aromatherapy
- Acupuncture
- Alexander Technique

Headaches

Headaches can be symptoms of an overstretched nervous system due to stress and exhaustion, but there are also other causes that need to be taken into consideration. For example, causes can also be related to the menstrual cycle, allergies, high and low blood pressure, digestive problems, low blood sugar, eye strain, poor posture, and back problems. It is important to find out the cause, especially if the headaches are chronic.

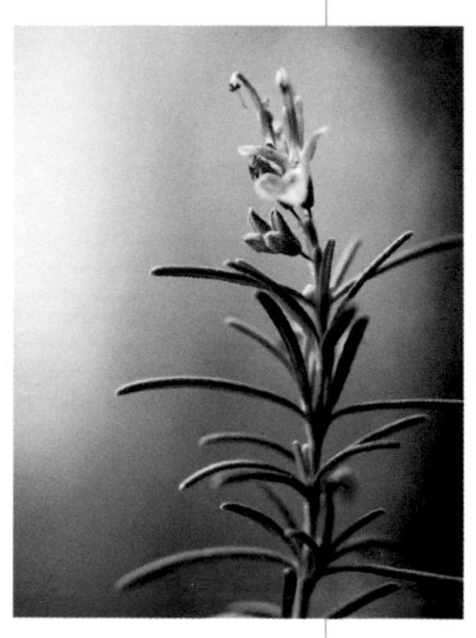

Above Rosemary has been used as a natural migraine treatment for centuries in Europe and China.

Herbal Pain Relief Herbal treatment for pain relief includes many herbs that have a wide range of associated actions. Consult the Herbal Directory (see pp.164–215) to find the herbs best suited to an individual. Suggestions include camomile, chrysanthemum (*ju hua*), feverfew, lavender, lemon balm, lime flower, passionflower, rosemary, skullcap, St. John's wort, and valerian. Choose several herbs in combination or on their own to make an infusion or decoction (see Herbal Methods section, pp.20–47), and drink as needed to ease the headache. Herbal baths using lavender, rosemary, or peppermint may also help.

Tension Headaches

Rosemary, crampbark, and valerian relieve the neck and shoulder tension that sometimes accompany a headache. If stress and anxiety are involved, use infusions of vervain, camomile, skullcap, and passionflower to calm and strengthen the nervous system and ease the pain. Drink as a tea when needed.

Migraines

These are intense headaches often accompanied with symptoms of nausea and vomiting. Visual disturbances can be early-warning signs that a migraine might be about to begin. Dizziness and light sensitivity indicate that the best treatment is to lie down and rest in a dark room.

Studies have shown that in most cases migraines can be aggravated by dietary factors, stress, hormonal imbalances, or structural problems. Allergic reactions to certain foods—the most common of which are red meat, chocolate, hard cheeses, coffee, and red wine—can trigger migraines. Stressful situations can also be a trigger for migraines, although many sufferers cope well while the pressure is on them only to find that the migraine returns when they relax. Migraines related to hormonal imbalances will occur regularly throughout each month with changes in the menstrual cycle. See other sections of the book to find herbal advice to strengthen the digestion, calm and relax the nerves, and balance the hormones. Osteopathic or chiropractic treatment is necessary to check and treat any structural problems concerning the head, neck, and spine.

Herbal Treatment An invaluable herb for migraine treatment is feverfew, which needs to be taken daily as a tablet or tea for at least a month before its effectiveness can be seen. Passionflower, willow bark, and valerian taken as a decoction or tincture at the first sign of pain may help to prevent the migraine from becoming too severe. Continue with a small dose of herbal medicine every few hours until the headache clears. To help ease digestive symptoms such as nausea and vomiting, sip cups of either peppermint, camomile, or meadowsweet tea.

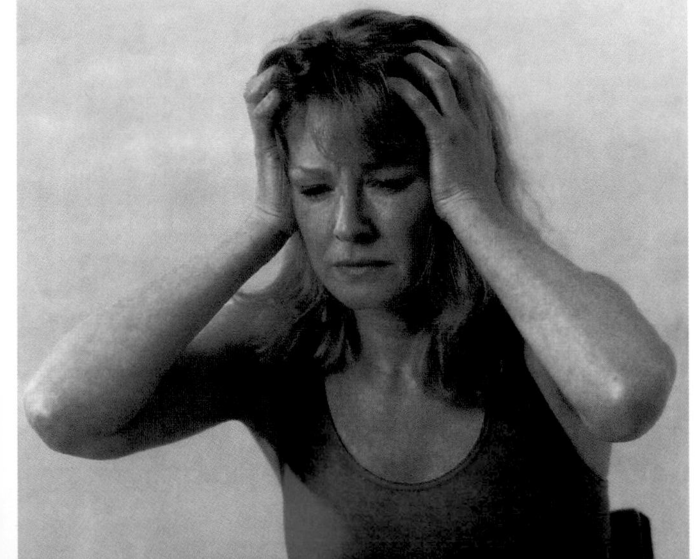

Left It is important to find out the cause of headaches, especially if they are chronic.

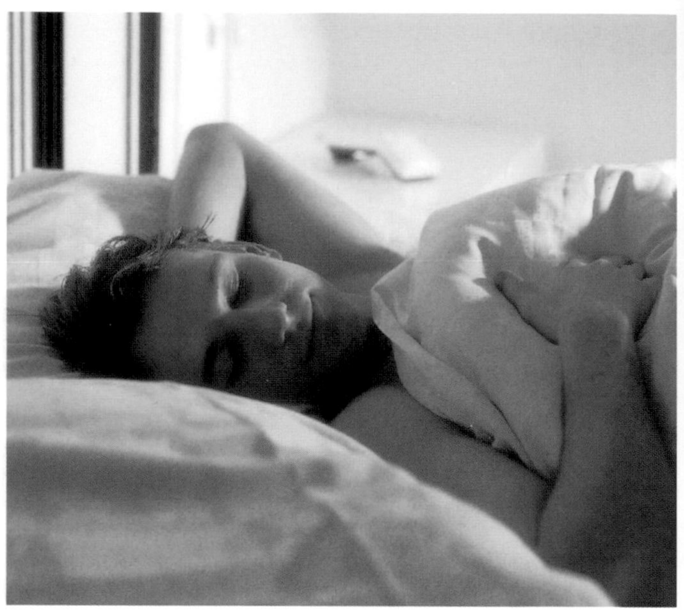

Right Rest is essential to relieve nervous exhaustion, which can result from long-term stress and anxiety.

Neuralgia

Nerve pain, or neuralgia, can be an excruciating pain that follows the path of a nerve, or a more localized pain where the nerve reaches the skin. Sciatica and facial neuralgia are both common types of nerve pain. They can be caused by a structural problem that may need osteopathic or chiropractic treatment. Generally there is some debility, and this is why the nerve pain and inflammation does not go away. Include lots of green vegetables and fruit in your diet, with extra supplements of vitamin B-complex for a while. Rest and relax to allow the body to heal itself.

Herbal Treatment This should include infusions, decoctions, or tinctures of ginseng, hops, passionflower, St. John's wort, and valerian. Choose the herb that suits your overall complaint and take it three times a day. Lavender and St. John's wort oil can be rubbed into the painful area, giving temporary relief from pain. If the neuralgia is associated with shingles, then take a tea or tincture of echinacea and calendula for a period of three months to cleanse and heal the body.

Nervous Exhaustion

Long-term stress and anxiety, overwork, insomnia, and poor diet may lead to low vitality and nervous exhaustion. During stressful periods, vitamins and minerals are used by the body in higher concentrations. It is often more difficult to eat well during these times. Greater amounts of tea, coffee, and alcohol may be consumed, all of which further deplete the body. This may create a destructive cycle where the energy is not being replenished, and there is little left to cope with the difficult situation. If nervous exhaustion reaches an extreme level, a collapse or breakdown occurs, which then forces rest and recovery. Rest, vitamin supplements of B-complex and C, and herbal treatment will help assist recovery of vitality.

Western Herbal Treatment Use a tea of red clover, dandelion leaves, and burdock to help cleanse the body, especially if large amounts of coffee, tea, and alcohol have been consumed. Nettles can help to tonify and remineralize the system. Nervine tonics such as oats, vervain, and skullcap will strengthen the nervous system. Drink these herbs three times a day, and avoid coffee, alcohol, and tobacco. Add licorice root to support their effect on the adrenal glands, which are often weakened by overwork and overconsumption of caffeine.

Chinese Herbal Treatment The Chinese herbs ginseng and astragalus will help to boost the physical energy as well as having a calming effect. Take one of them as a Chinese herbal decoction twice a day.

The Immune System

The immune system keeps us healthy by fighting off the many organisms that attack the body, including bacteria, viruses, fungi, parasites, and allergens. It is a complex system that is well integrated into all aspects of the body and has many levels of defense.

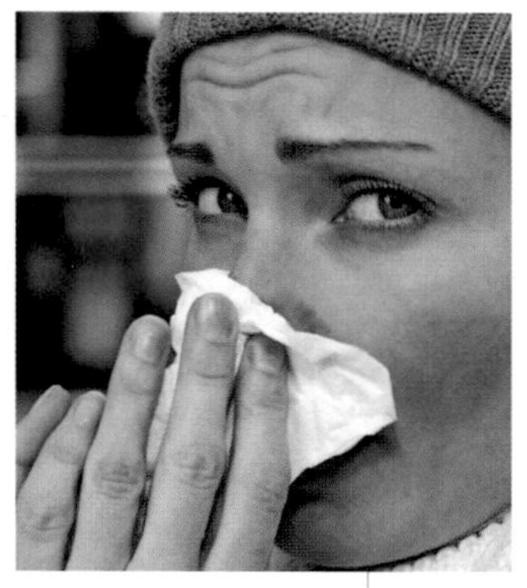

Above A strong immune system is needed to ward off colds and viruses,

The body has many intricate mechanisms to fight off potentially harmful microorganisms. Tears and saliva are antiseptic; the nose and chest have tiny hairs and sticky mucus in which to trap organisms; and the skin is coated in a protective oil. To get rid of harmful organisms, the stomach and vagina contain acids; the bladder flushes such organisms out; and the bowels contain gut flora that helps clear them. The blood contains white blood cells which attack an infection. If these natural systems fail, the lymphatic system is put into action and antibodies are produced to fight the invading micoorganisms.

The Role of the Lymphatic System

The lymphatic system is a network of tiny vessels that carry lymph, a colorless liquid that picks up debris and microorganisms, and lymph nodes, which are concentrations of white blood cells. The lymph nodes are situated in groups in the neck, armpits, groin, chest, and abdomen. White blood cells consume the harmful microbes and filter out debris. They also produce antibodies, which are carried throughout the body via the lymph. When the body is under attack, the lymph nodes swell and feel tender.

Interaction with the Body

The immune system is integrated into the body as described above. A healthy diet and good digestion are important in the production of lymph. Lymph is moved throughout the body by the contractions of the muscles. The liver is the main detoxifying organ in the body, and the debris from infections is filtered out from the blood.

How the Immune System Works

The blood capillaries are impermeable to large molecules such as proteins. Any protein that leaks into the tissue fluid from cells or plasma cannot therefore enter the bloodstream. These molecules are absorbed, along with some tissue fluid, by the lymphatic system.

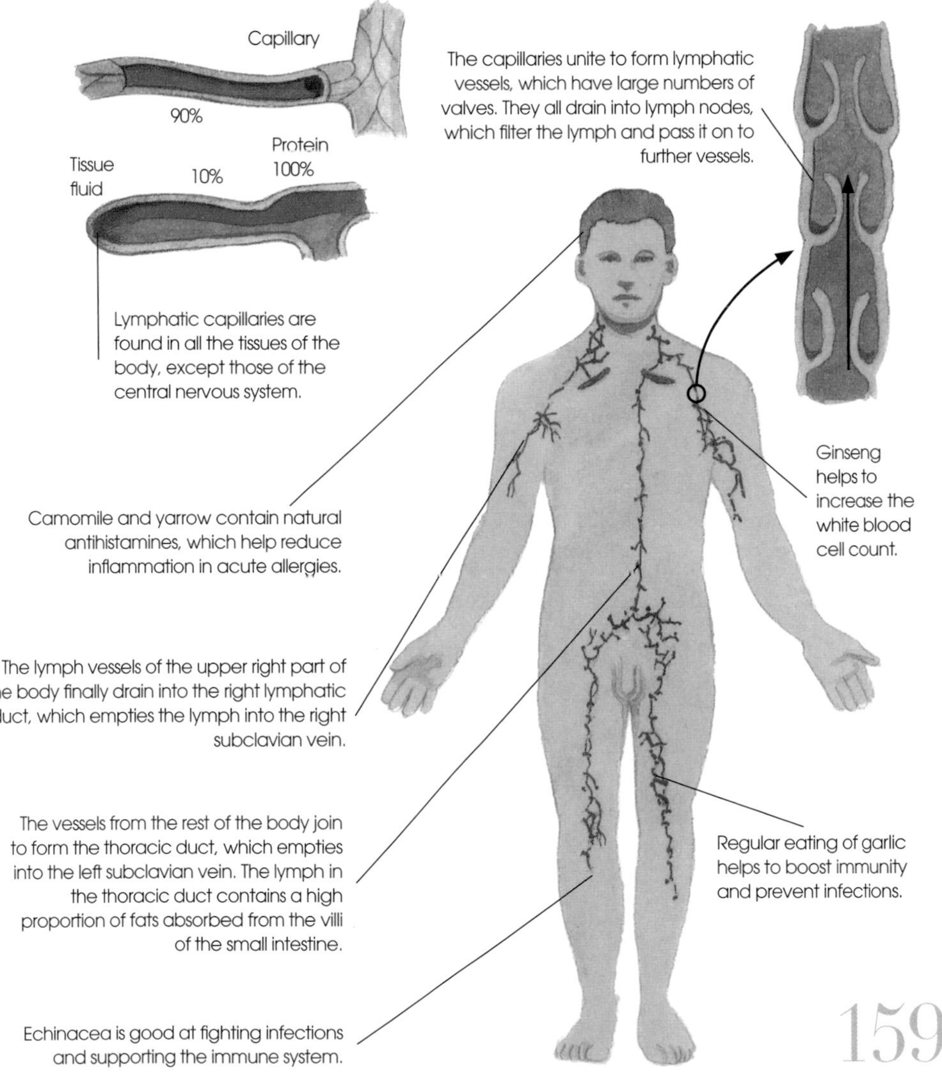

Capillary
90%
Protein
100%
Tissue
fluid
10%
The capillaries unite to form lymphatic vessels, which have large numbers of valves. They all drain into lymph nodes, which filter the lymph and pass it on to further vessels.
Lymphatic capillaries are found in all the tissues of the body, except those of the central nervous system.
Ginseng helps to increase the white blood cell count.
Camomile and yarrow contain natural antihistamines, which help reduce inflammation in acute allergies.
The lymph vessels of the upper right part of the body finally drain into the right lymphatic duct, which empties the lymph into the right subclavian vein.
The vessels from the rest of the body join to form the thoracic duct, which empties into the left subclavian vein. The lymph in the thoracic duct contains a high proportion of fats absorbed from the villi of the small intestine.
Regular eating of garlic helps to boost immunity and prevent infections.
Echinacea is good at fighting infections and supporting the immune system.

The Chinese Medicine Approach

In traditional Chinese medicine, the immune system is regarded as the *wei qi*, or defensive energy, that surrounds the body. It is closely related to the digestive system, and herbs that strengthen this, such as ginseng and astragalus (*huang qi*), help to build up this energy. If the *wei qi* is strong, infections are prevented from taking hold in the body.

Boosting Immunity

There are several factors that impair the immune system and weaken it. Stress, a poor diet and nutritional deficiencies, environmental pollution, injury and surgery, digestive problems, and the over-use of antibiotics can all impair the immune system. A positive and relaxed state of mind will help to increase the body's ability to cope with allergies and disease. A wholefood diet high in organic fruits and vegetables, nuts, beans and pulses, and unrefined oils will provide a good foundation for a healthy immune system. Using herbs that strengthen the immune system and help recovery from illness and injury, will enhance healthy functioning in all systems of the body.

Strengthening the Immune System

There are many herbs that will help to boost the immune system. Garlic is one of nature's best anti-microbial products that helps to prevent infections, even for those who have become immune to antibiotics. Take one or two garlic perles morning and night. Borage has a supportive and restorative effect on the adrenal glands. It is used to help with depression and other stress-related problems, as well as to aid convalescence. Wild yam has an anti-inflammatory effect, helping to relieve symptoms of infection and allergy. It is also a tonic for the digestive tract and liver. As an alternative to antibiotics, echinacea is useful for fighting infections and cleansing the blood and lymphatic system.

Chinese Herbs

Astragalus (*huang qi*) can be used to increase energy and build resistance to disease. Chinese angelica (*dang qui*) helps to restore energy and vitality, and stimulates white blood cell and antibody formation. Licorice (*gan cao*) can be taken during recovery from illness, and helps to support the functions of the liver and adrenal glands; it also enhances the immune system by stimulating the formation of white blood cells and antibodies. Ginseng is a wonderful remedy which boosts immunity and energy and enables the body to cope with stress. It can increase the white blood cell count, and benefits the liver and spleen.

Ailments of the Immune System

In this section ailments related to a low immune system are discussed. Herbal and more conventional treatments for infections are reviewed. Suggestions are given to reduce the side-effects of antibiotics and other drugs. Ways of finding out and recognizing possible allergic substances, and treatment for allergies, are given.

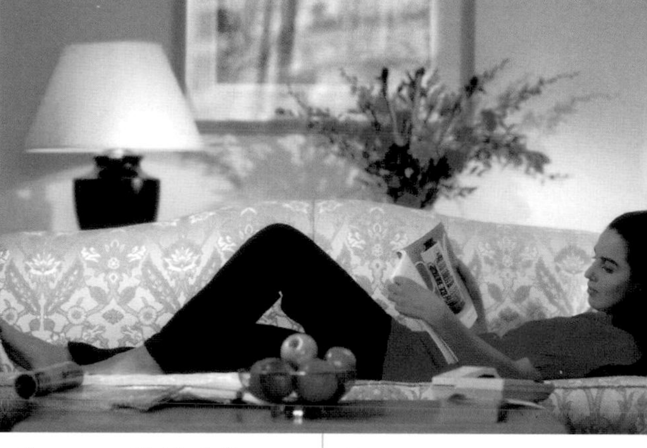

Above
Convalescence following an illness needs to include rest, a healthy diet, and herbal treatment to help boost immunity.

Infections

Bacterial and viral infections are the most common form of acute illnesses. Bacteria can invade the respiratory and the digestive systems, causing complaints such as throat, ear, and chest infections, and gastric upsets. Colds, influenza, and infectious diseases found in childhood are often due to viral infections. Supplements of vitamin C can be used to boost immunity. Take up to ¼ tsp (.5 g) three or four times a day. If this is more than the body needs, it will be excreted through the urine, and may cause diarrhea. Garlic will also help fight both viral and bacterial infections.

Antibiotics If there is a lot of pain or a high fever, antibiotics are a valuable tool in fighting bacterial infections, such as those of the inner ear, throat, or chest. If the body temperature goes above 104°F (40°C), or there are symptoms of confusion, or loss of consciousness, or twitching, you must consult a doctor immediately. If the fever or pain lasts for more than three days without signs of improvement, professional medical advice is needed. Antibiotics can be useful for

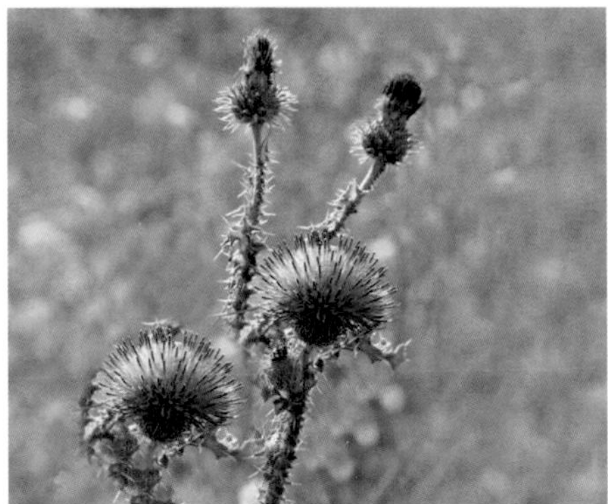

Above Milk thistle supports the function of the liver. It is especially useful in cases where long-term drug use may have caused damage.

infections that are not clearing with the use of other forms of treatment, particularly when the person is showing signs of weakening from the illness.

Dietary Factors If antibiotics are prescribed, herbal and dietary treatments can help prevent side-effects and boost the immune system to avoid repeated attacks of infections. Side-effects include gastric upsets such as constipation, diarrhea, and abdominal pain and bloating. Garlic can be taken to boost the immune system, to protect the liver, and prevent gastric disturbances. Eat live yogurt or take lactobacillus tablets (acidophilus) to protect the intestinal bacteria and eliminate toxins and harmful organisms via the bowel. Drink a glass of water with a teaspoon of cider vinegar daily to help clear the digestive tract. Drink plenty of water and urinate frequently to flush the toxins through the system, and help the kidneys and bowels with elimination.

Herbal Treatment The liver and the kidneys are involved in the filtering of toxins that are the result of drug therapy, including antibiotics. They are susceptible to stress from this process, and herbal treatment can be used to strengthen and support them. Chinese angelica, rosemary, and dandelion root can support the action of the liver and help it to break down toxins. Dandelion root, milk thistle, agrimony, and echinacea help to repair liver damage that may be caused by a long-term use of drugs. Celery seed will support the kidneys with the filtering and elimination of toxins. Take these herbs as teas or tinctures as needed (see Herbal Methods section, pp.20–47).

Allergies

An allergic reaction is caused when the immune system reacts against a substance that is not potentially infectious or harmful, but in fact may be nutritious and beneficial. The linings of mucus membranes in the digestive and respiratory tracts become inflamed and release a chemical called histamine. This can cause inflammation of the nasal passages, over-production of mucus, eye irritation, asthma, diarrhea, and urticaria (hives). Hayfever, asthma, eczema, bowel problems, migraines, and headaches can all be symptoms of allergic reactions.

Food Allergies

The most common food allergies are to wheat, dairy produce, eggs, oranges, tomatoes, peanuts, gluten (a protein found in oats, wheat, barley, and rye), food additives, and yeast. If a food allergy is suspected, remove one of the foods completely from the diet for two weeks. Sometimes the symptom of the allergy disappears within a few days. At other times it can take much longer and become worse before it gets better. Introduce the food back into the diet in a small amount every few days until it can be tolerated. Some allergies are for life, for example those related to strawberries, penicillin, and shellfish. It is possible to be allergic to more than one food or additive, so consult a qualified nutritionist to try out a complete food allergy elimination diet.

Herbal Treatment Combine echinacea, red clover, borage, and licorice and drink as a tea three times daily over several months to help boost the immune system. A tea of marshmallow and slippery elm before meals will soothe the digestive tract if there are symptoms of upset. Camomile or yarrow teas contain natural anti-histamines, and help to reduce inflammations in acute allergies; they can be taken frequently. Nettle tea or soup also helps to calm allergic responses, and is strengthening to the body.

Chinese Herbal Treatment The patent remedy *Bu Zhong Yi Qi Wan* (Central Qi Pills) contains the Chinese herbs ginseng, astragalus (*huang qi*), angelica (*dang gui)*, and licorice (*gan cao*). These herbs help to boost the immune system and strengthen the body, preventing allergic reactions from having their full effect. It is useful in the treatment of food allergies where symptoms affect the digestive system, combined with those of general signs of weakness, such as tiredness, a pale complexion, weak limbs, and shortness of breath.

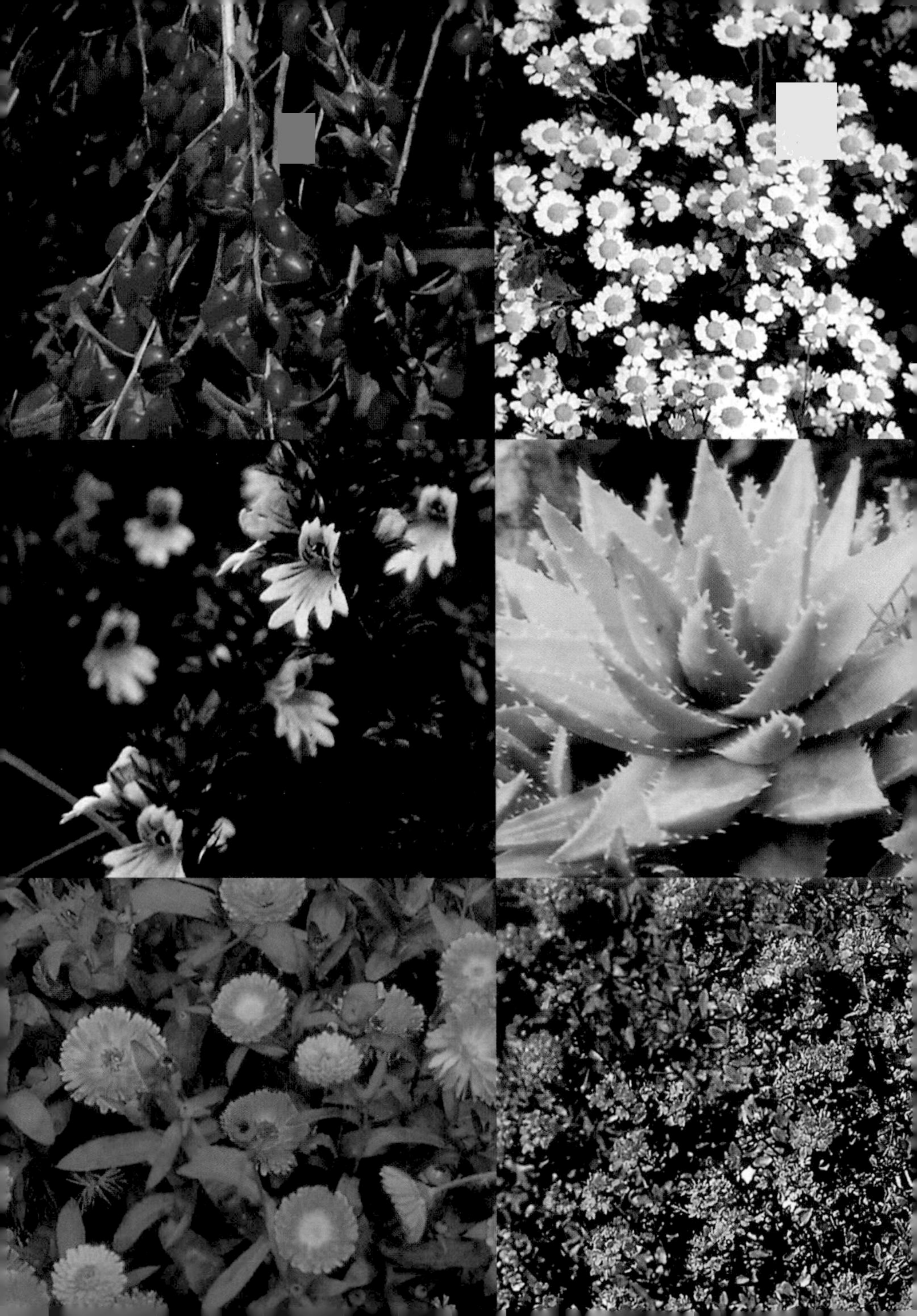

Herbal Directory

From *Achillea millefolium* to *Zingiber officinale*, this section provides information on the applications, methods of preparation, dosages and contraindications of fifty common herbs.

Yarrow

Compositae ACHILLEA MILLEFOLIUM

This herb is a native of Europe, naturalized in North America and grown in many other countries with a mild climate. The leaves are alternate, split into many fronds, while the flowers are white or pink.

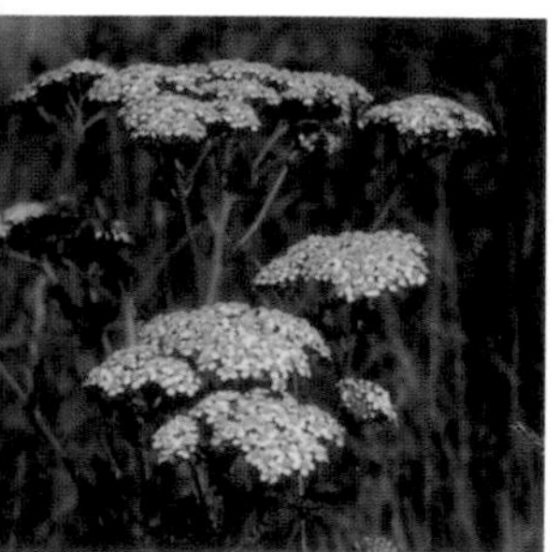

How it Works in the Body

- Pigenin has been shown to have anti-inflammatory and antispasmodic properties.
- The azulenes and salicylic acids are also both antispasmodic.
- The alkaloids have a hemostatic action, so help to stop bleeding.
- Chamazulene (as in camomile) is antiallergenic.
- It has a diaphoretic property (increases sweating).
- Useful as a tonic to promote digestion after illness.
- It has an antispasmodic and slightly diuretic action.
- A menstrual regulator, which helps to reduce heavy bleeding. Conversely, it can also bring on a period.

Parts used Herb.

Active constituents Volatile oil, containing salicylic acid and sesquiterpene lactones; plant acids; alkaloids; azulene, including chamazulene; and flavonoids including apigenin.

Applications

Tea Yarrow can be taken with other herbs (see Cold and Flu Tea, p.28) 8 fl oz (200 ml) three times daily.
Tincture Take 20 drops (1 ml) three times a day.

Indications

- Colds, flu, and fever.
- Allergies and hayfever.
- Indigestion, lack of appetite.
- High blood pressure.
- Varicose veins and other vascular problems.
- To regulate periods and reduce heavy periods.

Contraindications

- **Do not** use in pregnancy.
- In rare cases yarrow can cause an allergic reaction; if this occurs consult a practitioner.

Lady's Mantle

Rosaceae ALCHEMILLA VULGARIS

Lady's mantle grows to around 1 ft (30 cm) high, and is a native of Europe. The lobed leaves are soft, downy and arranged in a rosette from which the tiny yellow-green flowers rise on stalks.

How it Works in the Body

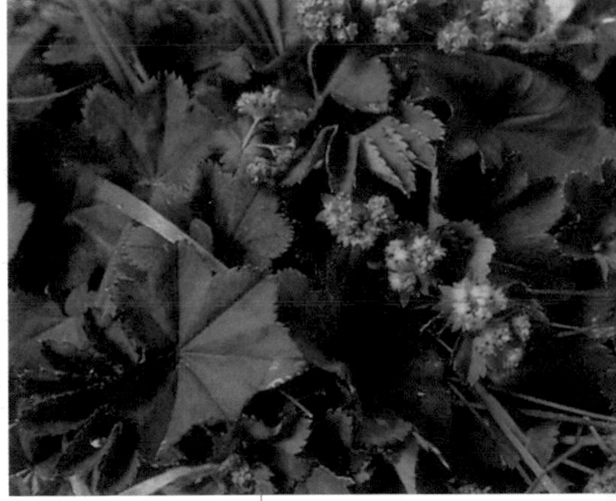

- The tannins act as an astringent, helping to reduce bleeding, particularly in the reproductive system.
- An excellent tonic for the uterus.
- The herb's properties enable it to act as a hormonal balancer, which also means that it has the effect of normalizing an irregular cycle.
- The salicylic acid acts as a mild painkiller.
- The protective layer the tannins form on the tissues means that this herb is also helpful in the digestive system.

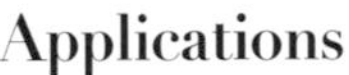

Applications

Infusion Use the leaves, 8 fl oz (200 ml), three times a day to help regularize the menstrual cycle and relieve heavy bleeding.
Tincture In stomach upsets where there is diarrhea, take the tincture, 40 drops (2 ml), three times a day.

Parts used Leaves and flowers.

Active constituents Tannins, salicylic acid.

Indications

- Heavy menstrual or menopausal bleeding.
- To help normalize an irregular menstrual cycle.
- Cramping pains associated with a period.
- Diarrhea in digestive disorders.

Contraindications

- **Do not** take this herb during pregnancy.

Garlic

Liliaceae ALLIUM SATIVUM

This plant is a member of the onion family and is cultivated all over the world for use in cooking as well as in medicines. The bulb is divided into cloves enveloped in a paper-like skin.

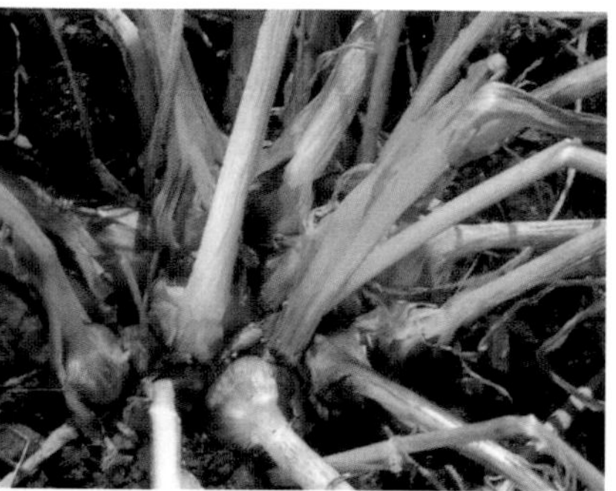

How it Works in the Body

- The volatile oil—which produces garlic's distinctive odor—contains allicin, which has an antibiotic effect on *staphylococcus aureus* and other bacterial infections.
- Allicin has also been effective against *candida albicans.*
- It has been shown to have a hypoglycemic effect, reducing blood sugar levels.
- Anti-thrombotic action reduces blood clotting, as well as lowering blood pressure and reducing cholesterol.

Applications

Salad dressing Use peeled, crushed cloves of fresh garlic in vinegar.
Cooking Use in cooking to benefit the immune system.
Syrup Take 1 tsp (5 ml) four or five times a day for sore throats.
Garlic juice, tablets and perles (capsules) are available commercially.

Parts used Bulb only.

Active constituents Volatile oil, including vitamins A, B, and C, allicin, enzymes, and flavonoids.

Indications

- Chest infections, including bronchitic ailments.
- Coughs, colds, and flu and to reduce catarrh.
- To reduce cholesterol, lower blood pressure, and to prevent thrombosis.
- Digestive problems.
- Late onset diabetes, to reduce blood sugar.
- May be taken alongside conventional antibiotics.

Contraindications

- **Do not** give raw garlic medicinally to children under 12.
- Only eat raw garlic with other foods.

Aloe Vera

Liliaceae ALOE VERA

Aloe vera, a succulent with long, fleshy leaves, originates from Africa but is now cultivated all over the world. It is often used as a house plant.

How it Works in the Body

- The properties of aloe vera mean that it is excellent as a vulnary or wound healer, mainly due to the anthraquinones in the clear aloe gel.
- It has a soothing quality when used on skin.
- The gel is good for the immune system.
- Bitter aloes have a laxative effect. Used in lower doses they will stimulate the colon, producing a bowel movement.
- Bitter aloes in larger doses act as a purgative, giving a much more vigorous action, which can result in griping pains.

Parts used Leaves contain two liquids: a clear gel that is used externally on the skin as a healing agent for cuts, scrapes, and burns; and "bitter aloes" from the rind , which act as a laxative when taken internally. *The "bitters" should never come into contact with the skin, and their use as a laxative should only be employed under the supervision of a practitioner.*

Active constituents
Polysaccharides, anthraquinone glycosides, known as "Aloin," and aloe-emodin, glycoproteins, saponins, and resins.

Application

Direct application to the skin The upper, fleshy parts of the leaves are broken off and split apart to release the clear gel. Apply the gel to the skin twice a day.

Indications

- First-aid remedy, to help heal cuts, scrapes, and grazes. Also useful for mild burns.
- To soothe itchy or dry skin.
- To help with digestive tract problems such as ulcers.

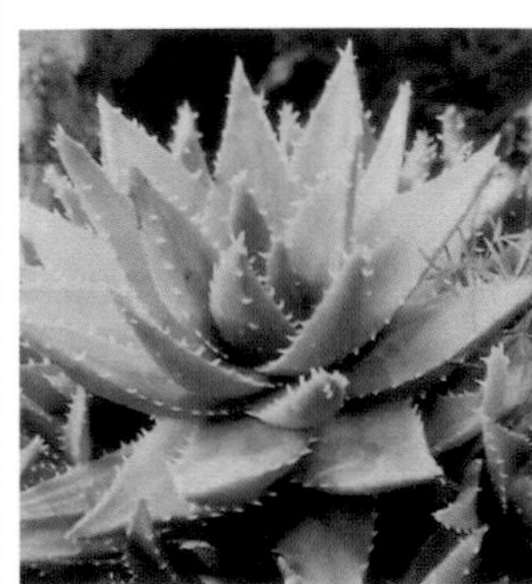

Contraindications

- Stimulates the uterus, so it **should never be used** during pregnancy or while breastfeeding.
- Avoid if suffering from kidney disease.

Marshmallow

Mavaceae ALTHAEA OFFICINALIS

This plant is native to Europe and is naturalized in North America. It grows to about 6 ft (2m), with pale-green, oval leaves covered in soft down, and white-pink flowers. The root is white.

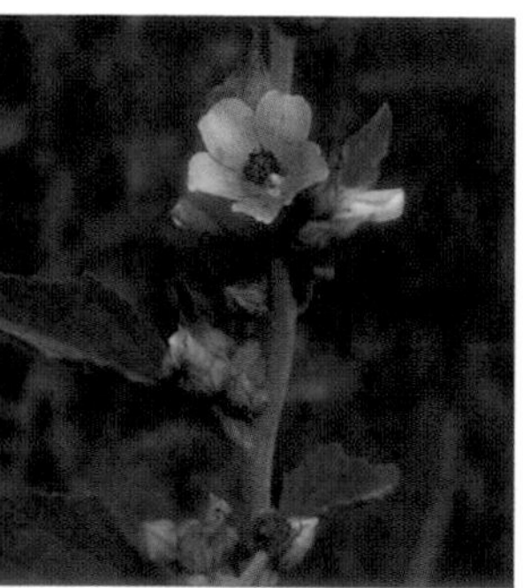

How it Works in the Body

- The mucilage is the main ingredient, which acts to soothe and protect tissues in the body:
- It is used to heal inflammation of the respiratory system.
- Heals inflammation of the digestive system.
- Used to calm irritated tissues in the urinary tract.
- Soothes and heals. It has been recommended as a poultice for skin problems.

Applications

Infusion of the flowers Take 8 fl oz (200 ml) three times daily. Externally, use the infusion as a wash for irritated skin.

Tincture Take 40 drops (2 ml), three times daily.

Poultice Can be used for boils or ulcerations, as well as a drawing paste or cream to treat insect stings, splinters, and boils.

Parts used Leaves, flowers, and roots.

Active constituents Root: mucilage 18–35 per cent, including polysaccharides, pectin, asparagine, tannins. Leaves: mucilage, flavonoids, coumarins, polyphenolic acids.

Indications

- Respiratory complaints, bronchitic complaints, and dry coughs.
- Digestion, including irritable bowel syndrome, diverticulitis, ulcers, and excess stomach acid.
- Urinary tract infections.
- As a wash for skin conditions.
- As a poultice for boils and ulcers.
- A drawing paste for stings and boils.

Contraindications

- None

Chinese Angelica

Umbelliferae ANGELICA SINENSIS *(dang gui)*

There are three main types of angelica: European, Chinese, and American. All three are helpful for the digestion and the circulation, but they cannot be used interchangeably.

Parts used Roots, rhizomes, leaves, stalks, and seeds.

Active constituents Volatile oil, coumarins, vitamin B12.

How it Works in the Body

- The variety described here has been selected for its wide-ranging applications. Chinese angelica's constituents make it especially useful for treating women's reproductive problems.
- Its combined action as a circulatory and blood tonic mean it is useful in menopause and to help with irregular and absent periods.
- Angelica's antispasmodic actions also help with painful periods.
- In China it is used to nourish the blood and prevent anemia, blurred vision, tinnitus, and palpitations.
- Like garden angelica it is a carminative herb for the digestion.
- The rhizome has an antibiotic quality and it is used for sores and abscesses.

Applications

Cooking Use the root in cooking as a tonic for circulation.
Wine Take one glass a day.
Infusion Take one or two cups daily. Dosage ⅛–¾ oz (3–15 g).

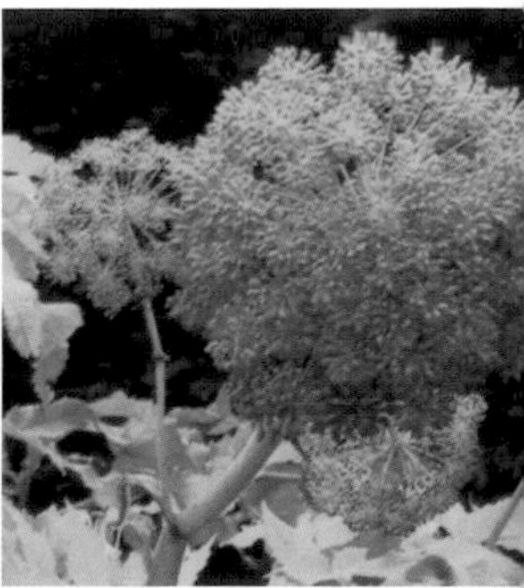

Indications

- Painful or irregular periods.
- Menopause, as a tonic for the reproductive system.
- As a circulatory herb for cold hands and feet.
- Improves digestion and eases constipation.
- Impaired liver function.

Contraindications

- **Do not** take during pregnancy.

Burdock

Compositae ARCTIUM LAPPA (*niu bang zi*)

Of European origin, this plant has also established itself in China and the United States. The burdock plant is from the thistle family and has large, broad leaves, and purple flowers with tiny hooks.

Parts used
Roots and leaves.

Active constituents In the leaves, sesquiterpenes, bitter glycosides, arctigenin, inulin, organic acids, and oils. Lignans, amino acids and polyacetylenes in the roots.

How it Works in the Body

- The plant's natural diuretic effect means it is mainly used is as an alterative or blood cleanser to remove waste products from the body.
- Used to treat rheumatic conditions.
- Lowers blood sugar levels.
- Arctigenin is effective at stimulating the liver.
- The fresh root has an antibiotic quality, probably due to the polyacetylenes.
- Stimulates digestion and aids appetite.

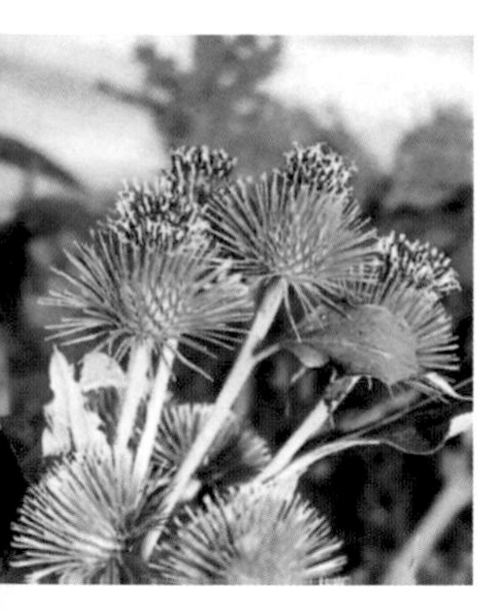

Applications

Decoction Use the roots with a liver herb such as dandelion. Take half a cup once a day.

Poultice Use the leaves for boils.

Tincture Use the leaves in a tincture for dry skin. Take for short periods only, 20 drops (1 ml) twice a day for up to four weeks.

Hair rinse The decoction can help with alopecia, or hair loss. The Chinese dosage is ⅛–½ oz (3–9 g).

Indications

- Infectious illnesses such as mumps and measles.
- Skin complaints, including eczema, psoriasis, acne, and boils.
- Arthritic conditions.
- Catarrh when there is a fever, cough, and sore throat.

Contraindications

- **Do not** use in pregnancy.

Mugwort

Compositae ARTEMISIA VULGARIS *(moxa-ail ye)*

This herb of European origin is also grown in China. The leaves are smooth green on the top and downy white underneath. Reddish-yellow flowers grow in spikes. It grows to about 3 ft (1m).

How it Works in the Body

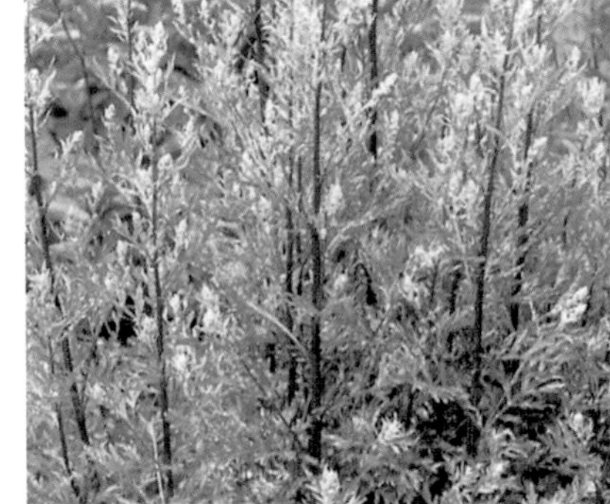

- Mugwort has been a traditional remedy for worms when taken in low dosage over a period of time.
- Can be used as a bitter, to increase appetite and promote digestion.
- Used to bring on menstruation.
- In Chinese medicine it is used to stop bleeding where the menstrual cycle is prolonged, and for uterine bleeding. It is also used for infertility due to a cold womb, and for menstrual pain.
- If used externally in the form of a *moxa* stick on specific acupuncture points, it can be used to help turn breech babies in the womb. Always seek medical guidance.

Applications

Tincture 20–40 drops (1–2 ml) twice daily.
Infusion Take 4 fl oz (100 ml) twice daily. In Chinese medicine the dosage is ⅛–½ oz (3–9 g).

Part used
Leaves.

Active constituents
Volatile oil, vulgarin (a sesquiterpene lactone), flavonoids, coumarin derivatives, triterpenes.

Indications

- Delayed or irregular periods.
- Loss of appetite, for example following illness.
- Sluggish digestion, especially for poor absorption.
- Increase bloodflow to injured muscles, aiding the healing of strains and sprains.

Contraindications

- **Do not** use in pregnancy.

Astragalus

Leguminosae ASTRAGALUS MEMBRANACEUS *(huang qi)*

Astragalus is a native of China, and while it is not so well known in the West its use is spreading. It grows to about 16 in (40 cm) high. The stems are hairy, and the leaves, up to fourteen of them, grow in pairs along them.

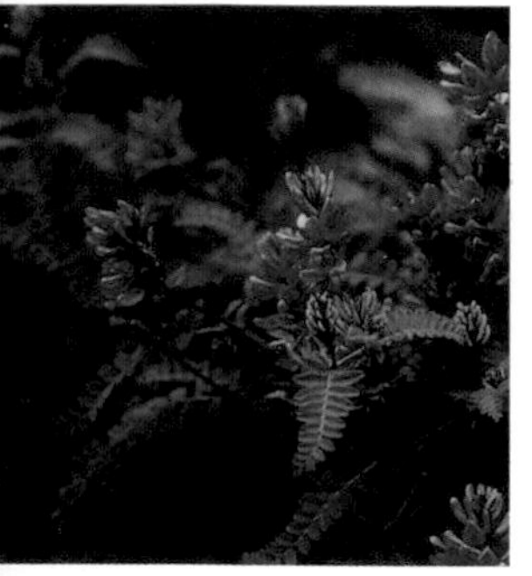

How it Works in the Body

- Astragalus is a stimulant to the immune system, and has a similar energizing effect to ginseng.
- Widely used as a diuretic for the urinary tract, and to reduce high blood pressure.
- Can help with water retention or edema.
- May be used with other herbs in cases of anemia.
- Used for excessive bleeding, for example during the menstrual cycle, and also after childbirth.
- Used externally as a wound healer.
- An aid to the digestive system.

Applications

Decoction One cup of astragalus may be taken twice daily.

Tincture Take 40 drops (2 ml) three times a day. The Chinese dosage is ½–1½ oz (9–30 g).

Parts used Root.

Active constituents
Asparagine, calcyosin, formononetin, astragalosides, kumatakenin, sterols.

Indications

- Water retention.
- High blood pressure.
- Colds and flu.
- Excessive menstrual bleeding and after childbirth.
- Ulcerative conditions and boils.
- Poor appetite and digestive weakness following illness.

Contraindications

- **Do not** take if you suffer from a skin disorder.

Marigold (Calendula)

Compositae CALENDULA OFFICINALIS

This garden plant grows to about 2 ft (60 cm). The flower resembles a large yellow or orange daisy and it has dark-green leaves. Native to Europe, it is cultivated in many other areas.

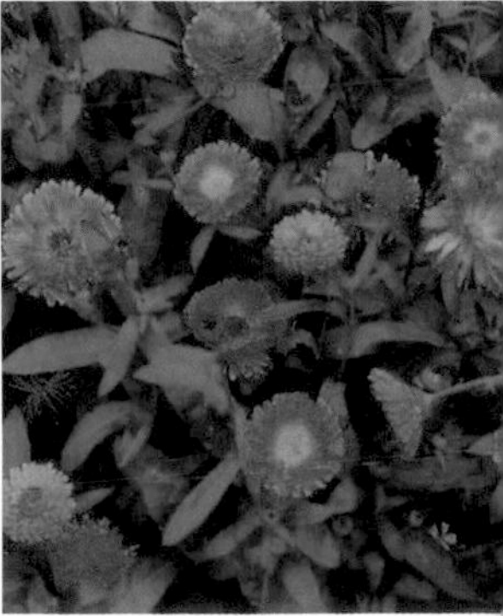

How it Works in the Body

- One of calendula's main actions is that of an antiseptic. This makes it especially valuable externally as a wound healer.
- Internally, it is beneficial to many skin disorders.
- It has a well-known antifungal action.
- Used for conditions such as varicose veins.
- Can help wth ulcerative conditions, digestive complaints, and as a liver tonic.
- Helps relieve menstrual symptoms.
- It is antibacterial and anti-viral.

Applications

Infusion Take 8 fl oz (200 ml), three times daily.

Tincture Take 40 drops (2 ml), twice a day.

Wash Use the infusion externally to clean cuts and scrapes.

Ointment Use on skin complaints or fungal infections.

Infused oil Apply to the skin to treat inflammation.

Indications

- Cuts, scrapes and wounds.
- Acne, eczema, psoriasis, and other inflammatory skin complaints.
- Diaper rash, sore and cracked nipples.
- Varicose veins.
- Fungal disorders, including *candida* (thrush).
- Stomach ulcers and gastric inflammation.

Contraindications

- None.

Parts used

Petals and flowerheads.

Active constituents

Triterpenes, including volatile oil, calendulosides, flavonoids, and chlorogenic acid.

Camomile

Compositae CHAMAEMELUM NOBILE/CHAMOMILLA RECUTITA

There are two types of camomile that are used medicinally, having broadly similar actions: Roman or garden camomile (*Chamaemelum nobile*), and German or wild camomile (*Chamomilla recutita*).

Parts used
Flowers and essential oil.

Active constituents
Volatile oil, principally chamazulene, flavonoids, sesquiterpene lactones, coumarins and phenolic acids.

How it Works in the Body

- Known as the "mother of the gut," its combined properties act as a muscle-relaxant in the gut.
- Calms and dispells nausea and indigestion.
- Works as a sedative for the nervous system.
- Effective as a cream or ointment for skin problems.
- It has an antiallergenic quality.

Applications

Infusion Add to baths to relax and calm.
Inhalation Useful for catarrh.
Ointment Use once or twice daily. Use as a poultice for slow-healing wounds, and as an eyewash to relieve tired eyes.
Tincture May be taken internally, up to 1 tsp (5 ml) three times a day if required, or 1 tsp (5 ml) at night to aid sleep.
Essential Oil Should only be used externally in a base oil for massage, or in a diffuser.

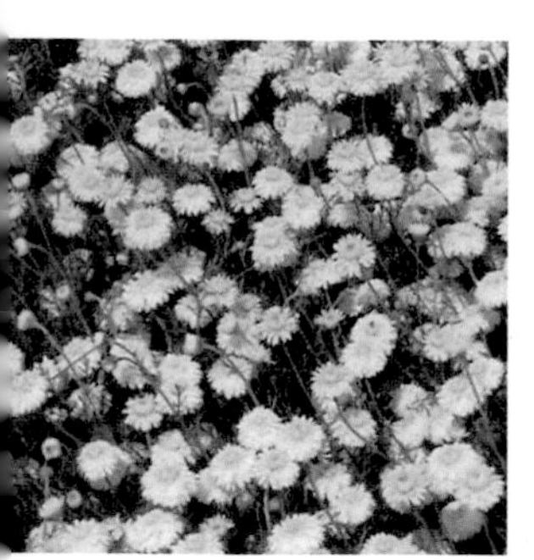

Indications

- Indigestion, wind, excess acid, and stomach ulcers. Used in nausea, especially in pregnancy, and for travel sickness, together with ginger.
- Aids restful sleep and relieve stress, tension, and headaches.
- Respiratory complaints, such as catarrh.
- Allergic conditions such as eczema, asthma, and hayfever.
- Topically to soothe dry and itching skin.
- For tired eyes—use in an eyebath.

Contraindications

- **Do not** use the essential oil internally or externally during pregnancy.

Chrysanthemum

Compositae CHRYSANTHEMUM MORIFOLIUM *(ju hua)*

This plant grows to just over 5 ft (1.5 m) high and is known in the West as "florist's chrysanthemum", as it is popularly used for flower displays.

How it Works in the Body

- Research has shown that chrysanthemum has an antibiotic principle, which is effective in laboratory conditions against *staphylococcus* and *streptococcus* bacteria, and so is a valuable remedy against infection.
- Yellow chrysanthemum acts on headache and eye problems.
- May reduce symptoms of hypertension and/or atherosclerosis.
- Helps to clear fever and headaches associated with colds and flu.
- Has long been used as a tonic for the eyes, especially where they are red, painful, and dry, or where there is excessive watering.
- Used also for spots in front of the eyes, blurry vision, or dizziness.

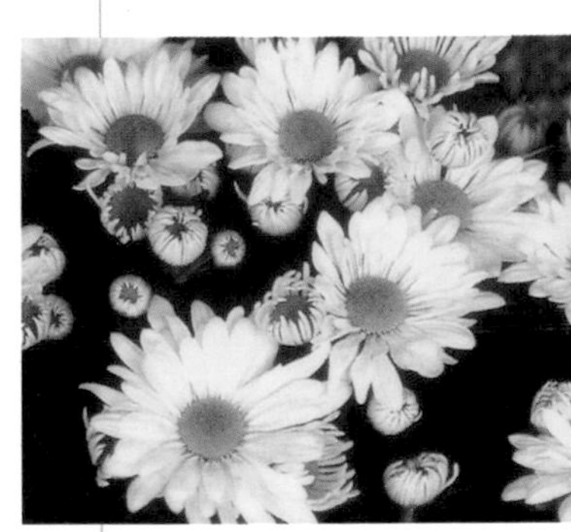

Applications

Infusion 8 fl oz (200 ml), taken three times a day.

Indications

- General conditions of infection.
- High blood pressure and related symptoms.
- Colds and flu accompanied by fever and headaches.
- As an eye tonic.

Contraindications

Do not take if you suffer from:

- *Qi* (energy) deficiencies.
- Weakness or poor appetite.
- Diarrhea.

Parts used
Flowering tops.

Active constituents
Alkaloids, volatile oil, sesquiterpene lactones, flavonoids, adenine, choline, stachydrine, chrysanthemin, and vitamin B1.

Black Cohosh

Ranunculaceae CIMICIFUGA RACEMOSA

A native American herb, it is traditionally used for women's complaints. It grows in Canada, the United States, and Europe. It has white flowers with toothed leaves and is noted for its black root.

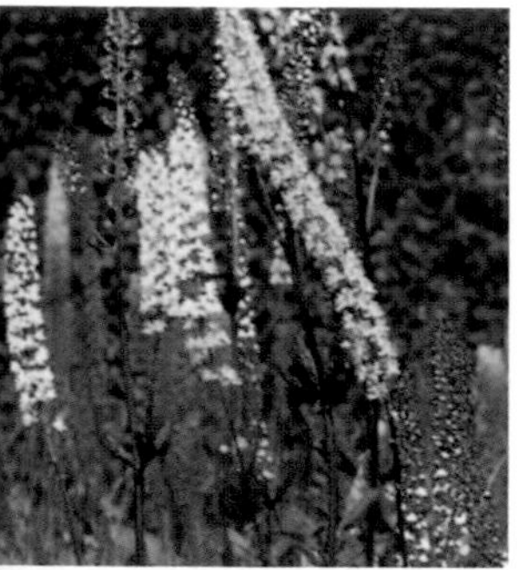

How it Works in the Body

- In North America, it is thought that black cohosh balances estrogen by stabilizing it.
- In European herbalism it is thought to have an estrogenic action, which actively works to reduce progesterone and promote estrogen.
- Used as an anti-inflammatory in arthritic conditions.
- Its sedative qualities have applications in other systems, for example, in lowering blood pressure, in reducing spasm and tension, and in the respiratory system.

Applications

This remedy is quite strong. Take care not to exceed the stated limits.

Decoction The root should only be taken in half-cupfuls, 4 fl oz (100 ml), twice a day.

Tincture May be taken 1 ml (20 drops), three times a day.

Parts used

Roots and rhizome.

Active constituents

Triterpene glycosides, isoflavones, isoferulic acid, volatile oil, and tannins.

Indications

- Period pains and cramp.
- Gynecological conditions where there is a lack of estrogen or an excess of progesterone.
- High blood pressure.
- Menopausal symptoms.
- Rheumatic complaints.
- Respiratory complaints such as asthma, bronchitis, and whooping cough.

Contraindications

- **Do not** take in pregnancy or while breastfeeding.
- **Do not** use where there is low blood pressure.

Hawthorn

Rosaceae CRATAEGUS MONOGYNA/CRATAEGUS OXYCANTHOIDES

Found in Europe, Africa, and Asia, the leaves are deeply lobed, and the flowers are white in the summer, giving way to bright-red berries in the fall.

How it Works in the Body

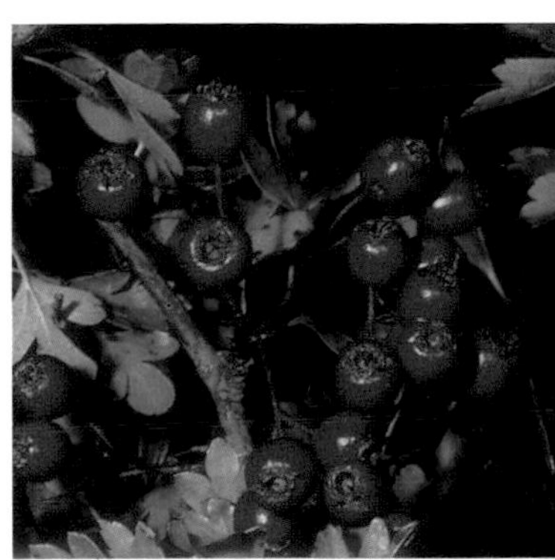

- Hawthorn acts on the cardiovascular system, regulating the heartbeat, relaxing the arteries and normalizing blood pressure.
- Used in angina and coronary artery disease to improve the blood flow to the heart muscles. Its effects are not instant, but taken over a period of months hawthorn can act as a tonic to the heart.
- Widely used as an aid to the digestive system, especially aiding the digestion of meat and greasy foods and relieving symptoms such as distension and diarrhea.

Applications

Infusion Of the flowers, leaves, or berries may be taken, 8 fl oz (200 ml), three times a day on a long-term basis.

Tincture May be taken 40–60 drops (2–3 ml), twice a day. There are no adverse effects from long-term use, and discontinuing use will produce no ill-effects.

Parts used

Flowers, leaves, and berries.

Active constituents

Amines (flowers only), flavonoids, phenolic acids, tannins, ascorbic acid.

Indications

- Symptoms of angina.
- Low or high blood pressure.
- Irregular heartbeat.
- Congestive heart failure and cardiomyopathy.

Contraindications

- Consult a doctor if you suffer from any cardiovascular condition.
- Hawthorn should not be taken if you suffer from acid regurgitation.

Purple Cone Flower

Compositae ECHINACEA PURPUREA/ANGUSTIFOLIA

Native to North America, the purple cone flower is cultivated in Europe and elsewhere. The flower is shaped like a daisy, with a ring of purple florets around a central cone.

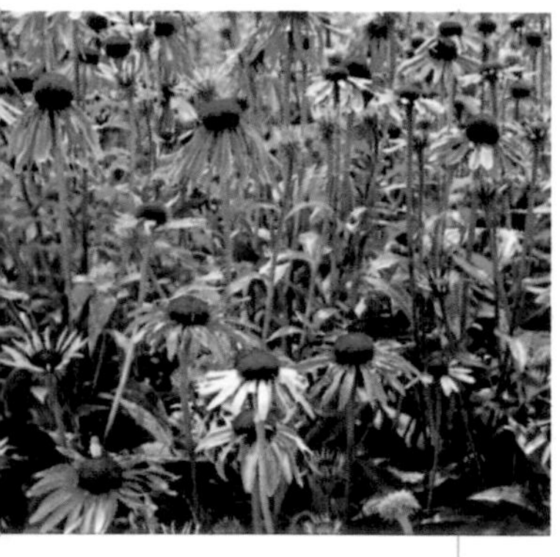

How it Works in the Body

- Polysaccharides play a key role in preventing viruses from taking hold in the body's cells, stimulating the white T-cells.
- Alkaloids perform an antibacterial and antifungal function.
- Can be used as an alterative, or blood cleanser.
- Aids the skin, clearing boils and other complaints.

Applications

Decoction of the root For infections, both viral and bacterial, take 8 fl oz (200 ml), twice a day.

Tincture Take 50 drops (2½ ml) three times a day. For sore throats and mouth ulcers, combine 40 drops (2 ml) of the tincture with 40 drops (2 ml) marigold tincture and 40 drops (2 ml) myrrh tincture in 4 fl oz (100 ml) water, and gargle three times a day.

Parts used
Root, rhizome.

Active constituents
Echinacoside (only in purpurea), isobutyl amides (including echinacin), polysaccharides, polyacetylenes, essential oil, alkaloids, and flavonoids.

Indications

- Colds, flu, sore throats.
- Chronic fatigue syndrome.
- Bacterial infections.
- Fungal infections such as *candida* (thrush).
- Skin complaints, including boils, acne, and eczema.
- Allergic conditions.

Contraindications

- Consult a doctor before taking if you suffer from HIV, AIDS or any other auto-immune disease.

Ginseng

Araliaceae ELEUTHEROCOCCUS SENTICOSUS *(ren shen)*

There are three main types of ginseng—Siberian, panax, and American. A native of Russia, China, Korea, and Japan, the bush grows to approximately 9 ft (3m). American ginseng is native to North America and the Himalayas.

How it Works in the Body

- Siberian ginseng is more stimulating than panax.
- American ginseng is similar to panax, but milder.
- Supports the adrenal glands to increase stamina and reduce lethargy.
- Relieves shock where there is loss of blood.
- Used for lack of appetite, chest and abdominal distension and chronic diarrhea.
- Benefits the heart, and helps palpitations with anxiety, insomnia, forgetfulness, and restlessness.

Parts used

Root.

Active constituents

Siberian ginseng: saponins, including eleutherosides A–F, glycans, volatile oil and two acetylenic compounds.
Panax ginseng: saponin glycosides.
American ginseng: steroidal saponins.

Applications

Decoction of the root Take 4 fl oz (100 ml) twice a day.
Tincture 2 ml (40 drops) three times a day.
Tablets Available commercially. Use stated dosage.

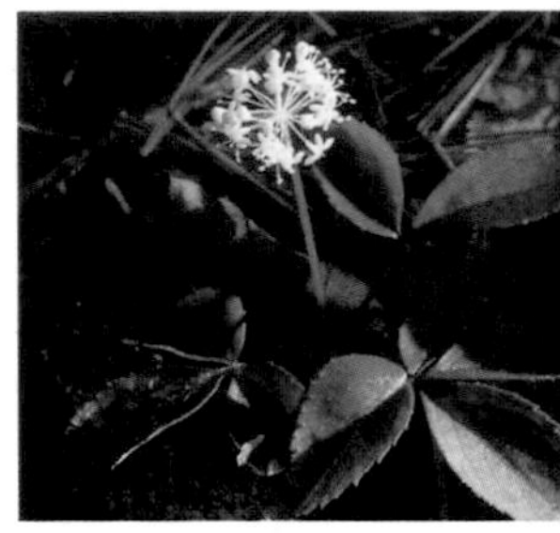

Indications

- Flu, colds, wheezing and shortness of breath.
- Viral illnesses.
- Emotional and physical stress including anxiety and insomnia.
- Male fertility problems (*Panax ginseng*).

Contraindications

- **Do not** take for longer than four weeks at a time.
- **Do not** combine with other energy stimulants.
- **Do not** take during preganancy.

Eyebright

Scrophulariaceae EUPHRASIA OFFICINALIS

Eyebright is one of a family of *Euphrasias* growing in Europe, Asia, and North America. It is a semiparasite, dependent on the roots of grass. The leaves are oval, and the flowers, appearing in summer, are white or lilac, shot through with purple veins.

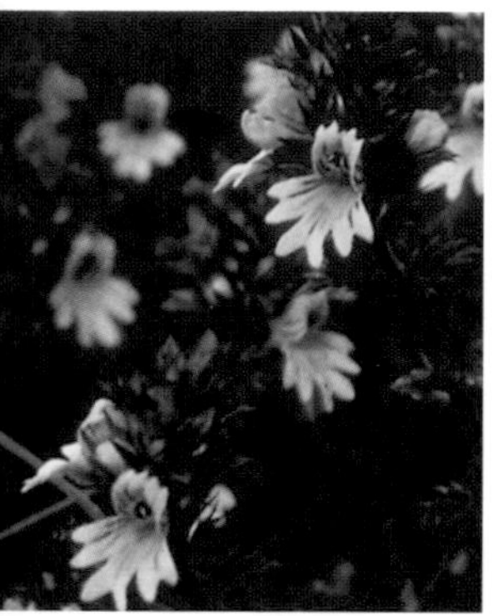

How it Works in the Body

- The astringent qualities found in eyebright form a protective layer on the mucus membranes of the eyes and reduces inflammation for infections such as conjunctivitis.
- Also helps to treat allergic conditions, such as streaming or irritated eyes as a result of hayfever or pollution.

Applications

Infusion Eyebright tea may be taken internally three times a day in order to counter infection or allergic conditions, especially where there is watering of the eyes.

Compress or eyewash For sore or irritated eyes. The eyewash should not be used more than twice a day. Follow the instructions in the Herbal Methods chapter (see pp.20–47) for preparations concerning the eyes.

Parts used
Whole herb.

Active constituents
Iridoid glycosides, tannins, phenolic acids, volatile oils, alkaloids, sterols.

Indications

- Infections or inflammations of the eye such as conjunctivitis and blepharitis.
- Allergic conditions including hayfever and allergic rhinitis.
- Tired or reddened eyes due to overwork, pollution, and tiredness.

Contraindications

- Seek further advice from a qualified herbal or medical practitioner for any eye condition that does not resolve in three to four days.
- Seek medical help immediately for any sudden pain or loss of vision.

Meadowsweet

Rosaceae FILIPENDULA ULMARIA

Native to Europe and parts of Asia, this meadow plant is also naturalized in North America. It grows to about 5 ft (1½m). Its paired and toothed leaves are green on top and pale underneath, with clusters of creamy flowers and a delicious scent.

How it Works in the Body

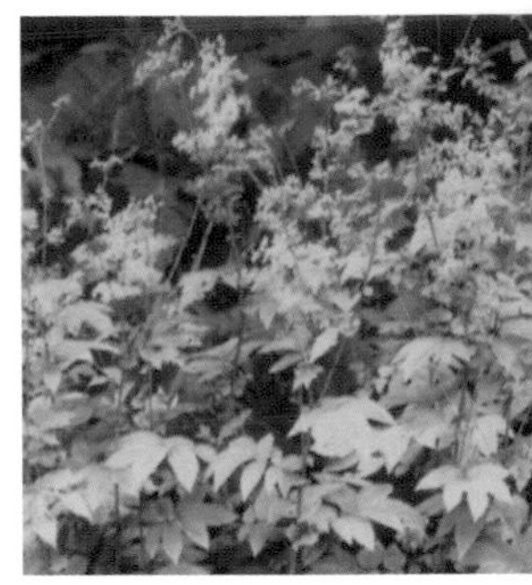

- The salicylic component in meadowsweet is responsible for the action of the plant as an anti-inflammatory and painkiller.
- Can be used in musculoskeletal disorders such as arthritis.
- It can be used where there is indigestion caused by the over-production of acid, for example to treat stomach ulcers or irritable bowel syndrome.
- It is not merely thought to reduce acidity, but to actively promote healing in the gut, where there is inflammation.
- Has long been used as a gentle remedy for diarrhea, and has a good reputation as a treatment for children's diarrhea.

Applications

Infusion 8 fl oz (200 ml) three times a day for digestive disorders. Use a double-strength infusion three times a day for diarrhea in adults.

Tincture 40 drops (2 ml) three times a day for arthritic complaints.

Parts used

Flowering herb, including leaves.

Active constituents

Volatile oil, with salicylaldehyde; phenolic glycosides, flavonoids, polyphenolics, tannins, coumarin, ascorbic acid.

Indications

- Digestive complaints, especially with acidity, for example, gastric ulcers, irritable bowel syndrome.
- Diarrhea in adults and children.
- Arthritic complaints.

Contraindications

- Meadowsweet should not be taken if you have an allergy to aspirin.
- **Do not** take if you have a sensitivity to salicylates.

Cleavers

Rubiaceae GALIUM APARINE

A garden weed found in Europe and North America. It has long, thin stems and whorls of leaves covered in tiny prickles that twine around other plants. The star-like flowers are tiny, white or greenish white.

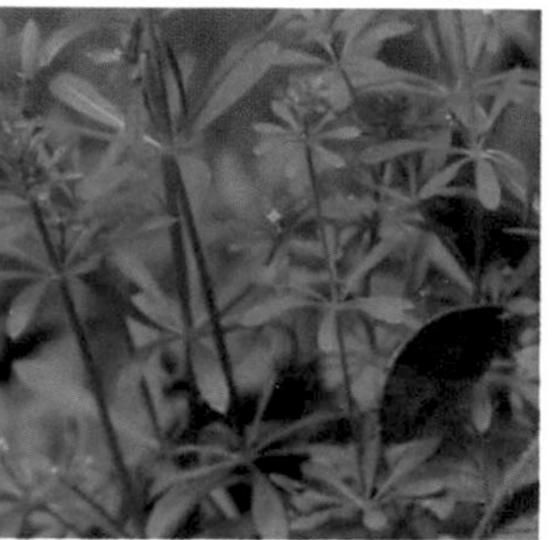

How it Works in the Body

- Cleavers' main action is that of a diuretic by eliminating toxins from the body via the urinary system.
- Helpful in skin conditions such as eczema and psoriasis.
- Effective as a lymphatic cleanser it can be used to treat swollen lymph glands.
- One of the iridoids acts as a mild laxative.
- Can be helpful to reduce blood pressure.
- For the nervous system it is used as a sleep tonic.

Applications

Juice Wash the fresh herb and add it with water to a food processor or blender to pulp it. Strain the juice and drink a wineglassful a day. It is possible to freeze the juice in icetrays and defrost as required.

Infusion Take 200 ml (8 fl oz), three times a day. Externally, the cooled infusion may be used as a wash or poultice for inflamed skin conditions.

Cream or ointment Useful for helping ulcers.

Parts used

Leaves and stems.

Active constituents

Iridoids, polyphenolic acids, anthraquinones (roots), alkanes and flavonoids, tannins and coumarins.

Indications

- Eczema and psoriasis.
- Ulcerations.
- Urinary tract complaints, such as kidney stones and cystitis.
- Insomnia.
- Swollen lymph glands.

Contraindications

- **Do not** use if you have low blood pressure.

Ginkgo

Ginkgoaceae GINKGO BILOBA *(bai guo)*

Also known as the maidenhair tree, ginkgo is a giant fern, native to China and Japan. It has one or more trunks, and the leaves are notable for their fan-like shape.

How it Works in the Body

- The ginkgolides, especially ginkgolide B, work as a platelet activating factor (PAF) antagonist.
- PAF is involved in initiating both allergic and inflammatory reactions, particularly asthma.
- The flavonoid portion is thought to improve circulation to the brain.

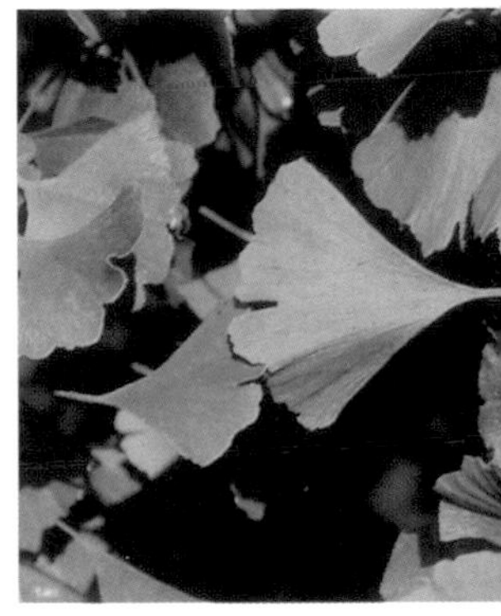

Applications

Infusion Prepared from leaves, take 8 fl oz (200 ml) twice a day.
Decoction Use the seeds. Take 8 fl oz (200 ml) twice a day.
Tincture prepared from the leaves. For circulatory problems take 1 tsp (5 ml), three times a day.

Indications

- Reduced memory, concentration.
- Age-related memory loss and dementia.
- Asthma, particularly in children (but be sure to only use under the guidance of a medical or herbal practitioner).

Parts used
Leaves and seeds.

Active constituents
Lignans; the ginkgolides (A, B and C), flavonoids, terpenes, essential oil, tannins.

Contraindications

- Consult an herbal or medical practitioner if you are already taking medication for a circulatory-related condition or asthma.
- Do not discontinue any medication.
- Exceeding the recommended dosage can cause headache, tremors, fever, or irritability. An effective antidote for excessive ginkgo consumption is 60 g (3 oz) of *Radix glycyrrhizae uralensis* (*gan cao*) or 30 g (1½ oz) of boiled ginkgo fruit shells.

Licorice

Leguminosae GLYCYRRHIZA GLABRA *(gan cao)*

Licorice has many different species. The roots have varying degrees of sweetness. Native of southern Europe and Asia, it grows to about 6 ft (2 m) and has pale-yellow flowers.

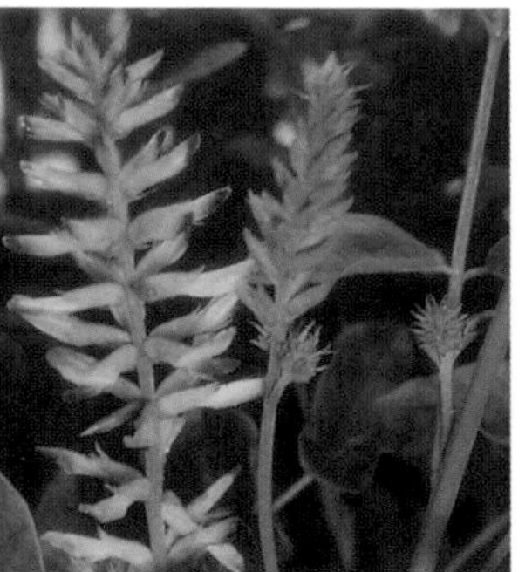

How it Works in the Body

- The glycyrrhizin acts as an expectorant (aiding hydration and secretion) and helping to prevent and ease coughing.
- Also works as an anti-inflammatory.
- Glycyrrhizin gives an antiallergenic effect, especially for asthma.
- It has a protective effect on the liver, and helps to detoxify the body.
- Used to treat nausea, bloating, vomiting and stomach ulcers.
- Can work as a laxative.
- Supports the adrenal glands in their function of healing the body.

Applications

Decoction 4 fl oz (100 ml) daily for constipation.

Tincture 40 drops (2 ml) twice a day. Make as a syrup to ease sore throats and dry coughs.

Mouthwash Use for mouth ulcers.

Parts used

Root.

Active constituents

Triterpenes (mainly glycyrrhizin), flavonoids and isoflavonoids, coumarins, chalcones, polysaccharides, volatile oil, starch, sugars.

Indications

- Bloating, nausea, indigestion and stomach ulcers.
- Mouth ulcers
- Mild asthma (seek the advie of a medical or herbal practitioner).
- Dry cough, chest complaints, bronchitic and catarrhal conditions
- Arthritis, where there are inflamed joints.

Contraindications

- **Do not** take during pregnancy.
- **Do not** take if suffering from high blood pressure.

Goldenseal

Ranunculaceae HYDRASTIS CANADENSIS

This herb from the buttercup family is a native of Canada and the eastern United States. The hairy stem leads to two lobed leaves and a small greenish-white flower. It has red fruit and a yellow root.

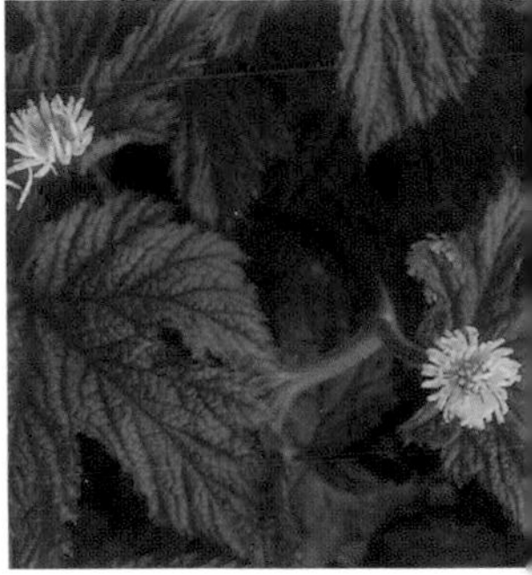

How it Works in the Body

- The isoquinoline alkaloids are thought to be largely responsible for goldenseal's medicinal actions, the hydrastine acting as an astringent and as a hemostatic agent (stops bleeding).
- Berberine has antibacterial and amoebicidal properties and canadine is thought to stimulate the uterine muscles.
- Its main use is in the treatment of the body's mucus membranes for conditions and infection of the eyes, nose, mouth and throat.
- Can increase appetite and stimulate digestion if used as a tonic.
- Alleviates heavy menstrual bleeding and vaginal infection.

Applications

Decoction Use as a gargle or mouthwash, two or three times a day.

Powder Prepare an infusion for use as a douche for vaginal infections.

Tincture 20 drops (1 ml), twice daily.

A dilute infusion May be used as an eyewash.

Indications

- Sore throat, sore gums, mouth ulcers.
- Inflamed or sore eyes.
- Loss of appetite.
- Constipation.
- Heavy menstrual bleeding and vaginal infection.

Contraindications

- **Do not** take in pregnancy or while breastfeeding.
- **Do not** take if you have high blood pressure.
- **Do not** exceed the dosages stated, goldenseal is toxic in large amounts.

Parts used

Rhizome.

Active constituents

Isoquinoline alkaloids (including hydrastine, berberine and canadine), fatty acids, resin, polyphenolic acids, volatile oil.

St. John's Wort

Hypericaceae HYPERICUM PERFOLIATUM

Native to Europe and Britain, and imported to North America. Grows to about 3 ft (1 m), it has small green leaves and bright-yellow flowers. The black dots on the underside of the petals are oil glands.

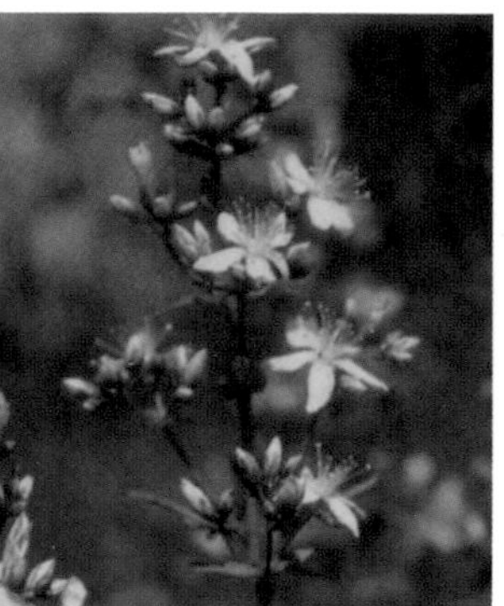

How it Works in the Body

- St. John's wort works primarily in the nervous system, the hypericin in combination with the other constituents acting as an antidepressant.
- Acts as a tonic for the nervous system as a whole.
- In the digestive system, the herb is beneficial to the liver.
- The anti-viral properties make it especially useful in colds and flu to boost the immune system.
- The oil is used as an antiseptic to heal wounds and to ease nerve pain, for example, in shingles and repetitive strain injury.

Applications

Infusion Take 8 fl oz (200 ml), twice a day.

Tincture Should be taken 40 drops (2 ml), three times a day. Externally, the oil may be applied twice a day (see nerve tonic oil, p.36).

Cream Apply twice a day to stings or cuts.

Parts used

Whole herb.

Active constituents

Essential oil, hypericins, flavonoids, and epicatechin.

Indications

- Mental or emotional stress or depression.
- Menopause associated with emotional debility.
- Digestive ailments.
- Colds and flu.
- Viral complaints, such as herpes, HIV, and AIDS.
- Shingles and repetitive strain injury.
- Stings or cuts.

Contraindications

- Do not exceed the stated dosage. Over-use of this herb can cause photosensitivity in some people.

Lavender

Labiatae LAVANDULA OFFICINALIS/ANGUSTIFOLIA

Native to the western Mediterranean, it is used in cosmetics for its fragrance. The leaves are narrow, gray-green, and the flowers form a pale- to dark-purple spike at the end of a tall stalk.

How it Works in the Body

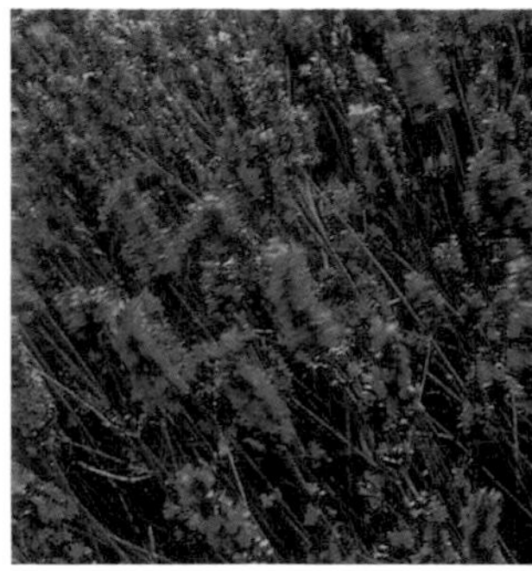

- Lavender has a calming and relaxing quality. It is suitable for use in the body's many systems.
- Helps calm indigestion, wind, and bloating.
- Relieves headaches, depression, and insomnia.
- Can be beneficial for asthmatics, where there is a nervous element contributing to the symptoms.
- It can be added to creams and oils as a rub to treat arthritic complaints and relieve painful joints.
- Cream or oil can help relieve symptoms of neuralgia or nerve pain.

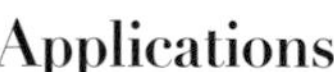

Applications

Infusion For indigestion, take 4 fl oz (100 ml).

Tincture For sleeplessness, take twice daily ½–1 tsp (3–5 ml).

Infusion or essential oil Add to a bath or use in a diffuser. Add two drops of essential oil to a bowl of cold water and soak a cloth to make a compress. Add five drops of oil to a footbath.

Rub Add one drop each of lavender and wintergreen essential oil to 4 tbsp (50 ml) of a carrier oil.

Parts used
Flowers, essential oil.

Active constituents
Volatile oil, coumarins, triterpenes.

Indications

- Indigestion, wind, and bloating.
- Nervous complaints, including tension, headaches and insomnia.
- Arthritic complaints and neuralgia.
- Insect bites and stings.

Contraindications

- Do not add to a baby's bath as oils can be ingested from the hands.

Motherwort

Labiatae LEONURUS CARDIACA *(yi mu cao)*

A native of Europe, this plant grows to about 3 ft (1 m), with dull-green, hairy leaves, and clusters of pink flowers. It is naturalized in other countries, including the UK and North America. It grows mainly on wasteground, but is occasionally cultivated in gardens.

Parts used
Whole herb.

Active constituents
Iridoids, diterpenes, flavonoids, caffeic acid.

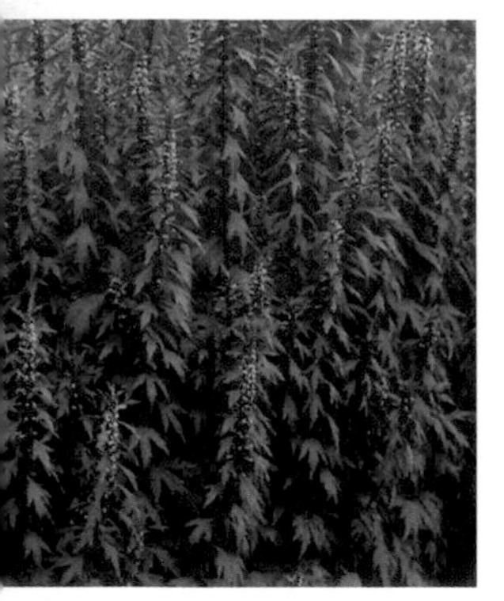

How it Works in the Body

- Motherwort is a remedy for the cardiovascular system, particularly where there are palpitations and when they are aggravated by nervous tension or stress.
- Its actions are antispasmodic and sedative, helping to regulate the heart, and also act as a tonic to strengthen weakness of the heart.
- Can be used to reduce symptoms of high blood pressure.
- Helps to bring on a delayed period by stimulating the muscles of the uterus.
- Also used where there is premenstrual syndrome, especially in early menopause.

Applications

Infusion 8 fl oz (200 ml) twice daily.
Tincture Take 40 drops (2 ml) three times a day.

Indications

- Palpitations associated with nervous tension and stress.
- Heart palpitations and weakness (always consult a doctor).
- High blood pressure.
- Premenstrual syndrome, especially in menopause.

Contraindications

- **Do not** take during pregnancy.
- **Do not** take when there is a tendency for heavy periods.

Honeysuckle

Caprifoliaceae LONICERA SPECIES *(jin yin hua)*

Honeysuckle is a European native, but is grown throughout the world. It is a climbing shrub, growing to some 12 ft (4 m) with oval leaves and yellow flowers either tinged with orange or white.

How it Works in the Body

Western applications of *Lonicera caprifolium* follow age-old usage:

- The leaves are used as a gargle or mouthwash for sore throats and gum problems.
- The flowers are commonly used in treatments for asthma, to relax the airways.
- Can help to protect the lungs in cases of tuberculosis.
- Also used in cases of damp-heat dysenteric disorders.
- Helps to soothe painful urinary dysfunction.

Parts used

Flowers and leaves.

Active constituents

Volatile oil, luteolin, inositol, tannins.

Applications

Infusion 8 fl oz (200 ml) twice daily, internally. Use the infusion as a gargle or mouthwash, twice daily (see Herbal Methods chapter, gargles and mouthwashes, p.32).

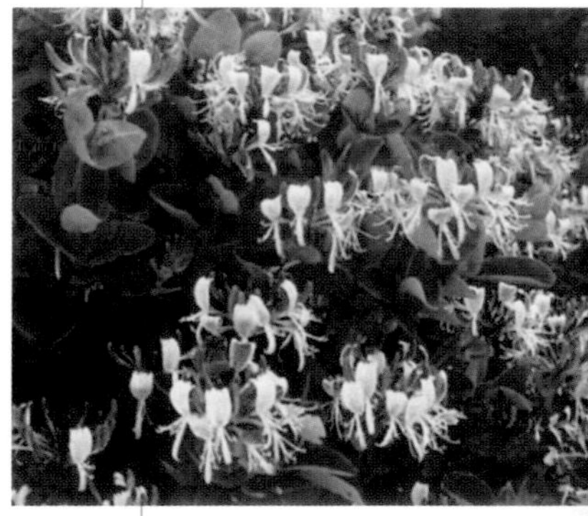

Indications

- Sore throat.
- Gum problems.
- Asthma (always consult a qualified herbal or medicinal practitioner).
- Infections accompanied by fever, sore throat, headache.
- Abscesses or swellings, especially if occuring in the breast or throat.
- Dysentery or painful urinary dysfunction.

Contraindications

- **Never** use the berries as they are poisonous.

Lycium Fruit

Solanaceae LYCIUM CHINENSE *(gou qi zi)*

This shrub is native to, and cultivated widely throughout, China. It grows to about 12 feet (4 m) and displays distinctive, bright-red berries.

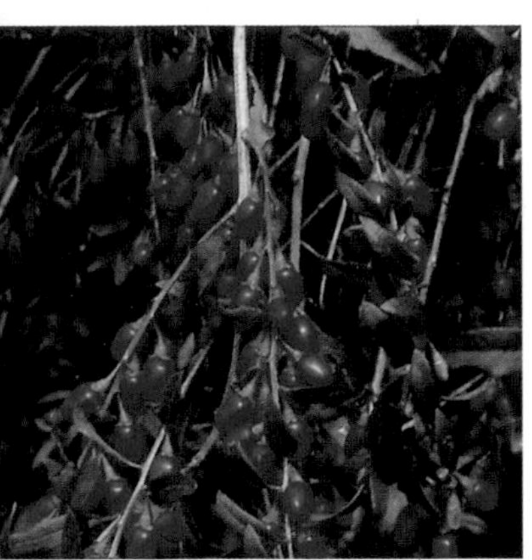

How it Works in the Body

- The berries are thought to have a protective effect on the liver and kidneys, nourishing them and acting as a tonic.
- Can be used to treat a range of ailments including pain in the back and legs, and low-grade abdominal pain.
- Helps to relieve diabetes and other wasting and thirsting disorders, including excessive urination at night (nocturia).
- Acts as a tonic for the eyes, especially where there is dizziness, blurred vision, and diminished sight.
- Can be used in the respiratory system as a tonic for the lungs.
- In the circulatory system, to reduce blood pressure and to lower lipid levels.

Parts used

Berries and root.

Active constituents

Betaine, carotene, physalien, thiamine, riboflavine, vitamin C, beta-sitosterol, and linoleic acid.

Applications

Decoction Use the berries and the root, take 8 fl oz (200 ml) a day.

Tincture Use the root, take 1 tsp (5 ml), twice daily.

Indications

- Liver and kidney ailments.
- High blood pressure and lipid levels.
- Diabetes.
- Consumptive coughs and respiratory ailments.
- Male impotence.

Contraindications

- Do not use in cases of digestive weakness or if you suffer from diarrhea.

Lemon Balm

Labiatae MELISSA OFFICINALIS

Common in Europe, Asia, North Africa, and North America, the oval leaves of lemon balm have serrated edges and when crushed they emit a lemon aroma. The flowers are white.

How it Works in the Body

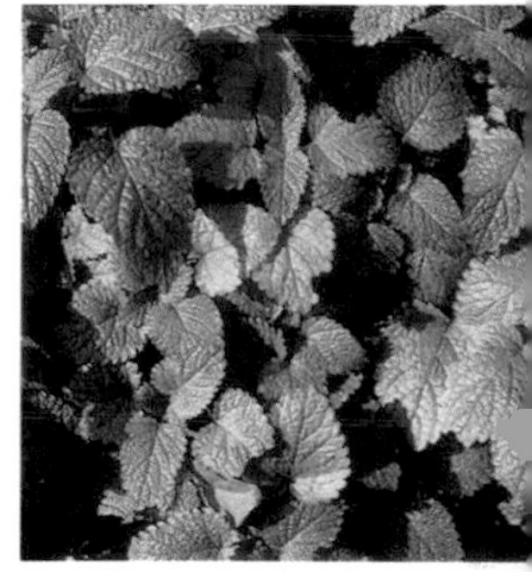

- The oil is the main agent used to calm and soothe the nervous system, and has a relaxing effect on the muscles. It can be used in states of excitability, palpitations, depression, and headache.
- The polyphenolics are responsible for an antiviral action: a cream made from lemon balm can be effective against cold sores.
- Lemon balm has also been used to help to treat an overactive thyroid by reducing the over-activity of the gland (hyperthyroidism).
- In the reproductive system, this herb has been used to ease symptoms of menopause, including hot flashes and anxiety.
- It is also used to regulate periods as well as to alleviate period pains.

Applications

Infusion 8 fl oz (200 ml) three times a day.
Tincture 60 drops (3 ml) twice a day.
Cream or ointment Use topically on cold sores (see Herbal Methods chapter, pp. 20–47).
Essential oil Use in an oil burner or add to a bath.

Parts used

Leaves and flowers, essential oil.

Active constituents

Volatile oil, flavonoids, polyphenolics (including rosmarinic acid, triterpenic acids).

Indications

- Nervous complaints.
- Viral complaints, such as cold sores, shingles, colds and flu.
- Menopause.
- Irregular or painful periods.

Contraindications

- Do not add to a baby's bath as the oils can be ingested from the hands.

Peppermint

Labiatae MENTHA PIPERITA *(bo he)*

A native of Europe, mint is perhaps one of the best-known culinary herbs. The medicinal variety is a hybrid—a naturally occurring combination of watermint and spearmint.

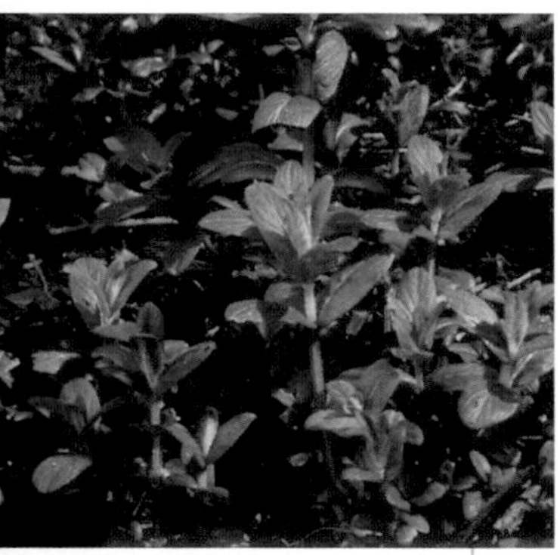

How it Works in the Body

- The menthol in the oil is responsible for an antiseptic effect on the body as a whole.
- The combination of constituents in the leaves has an antispasmodic effect, calming the gut, especially in an upset which is due to over-indulgence.
- Used in complaints such as irritable bowel syndrome, gastritis, and for excess wind and colic.
- Contains a diaphoretic element that encourages sweating, so can be used to cool down a fever resulting from cold or flu.

Applications

Infusion Take 8 fl oz (200 ml) three times a day after meals to aid digestion. Add a pinch of the herb to a tea made of equal parts of yarrow and elderflower to relieve symptoms of cold and flu.

Tincture 20 drops (1 ml), three times a day. Use 10 drops of the oil in 4 tbsp (50 ml) of carrier oil to rub onto inflamed joints.

Peppermint capsules are available on prescription.

Parts used

Leaves, essential oil.

Active constituents

Essential oil, up to 1.5 per cent, containing menthol, flavonoids, rosmarinic acid.

Indications

- Irritable bowel syndrome, gastritis, excess wind, and colic.
- Colds and flu.
- Inflamed joints.

Contraindications

- **Do not** ingest the oil, use on children or take when breastfeeding.

Passionflower

Passifloraceae PASSIFLORA INCARNATA

Passionflower is native to the southern United States and also to central and South America, and it cultivated in many other areas. It is a climber, of approximately 30 ft (9 m) in length.

How it Works in the Body

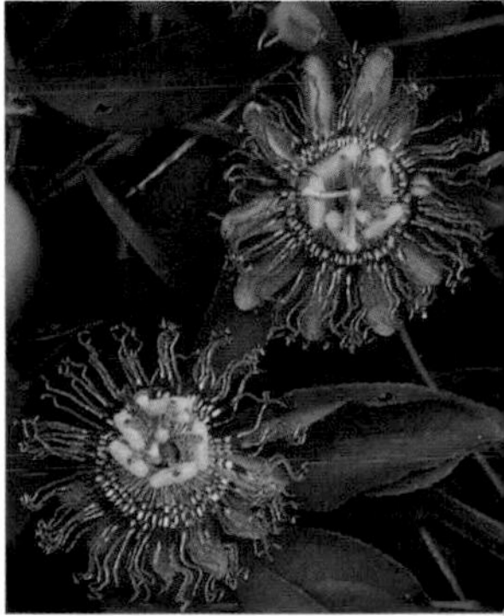

- Passiflora is primarily a sedative acting on the central nervous system, through the combined actions of the alkaloids, flavonoids, and the 8-pyrone derivative.
- The herb's sedative qualities have been used in overactive states ranging from epilepsy to neuralgia and anxiety.
- The flavonoid, apigenin, is known to have antispasmodic and anti-inflammatory action, which has been used to ease high blood pressure, quiet palpitations and to relieve muscle spasms.
- Useful in states of sleeplessness.

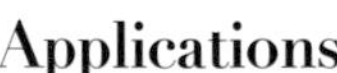

Applications

Infusion Take 8–16 fl oz (200–400 ml) daily.

Tincture Take 40 drops (2 ml) three times a day, or 1 tsp (5 ml) at night for insomnia.

Tablets Available commercially. Use stated dosage.

Indications

- Anxiety, restlessness, panic attacks.
- Insomnia.
- Neuralgia.
- High blood pressure.
- Diverticulitis.
- Irritable bowel syndrome.
- Period and ovarian pain.

Contraindications

- **Do not** use during pregnancy.
- Large doses can lead to a soporific state.

Parts used

Leaves.

Active constituents

Alkaloids (some of which have not been fully verified), flavonoids (including apigenin, an 8-pyrone derivative), sterols, and sugars.

Rosemary

Labiatae ROSMARINUS OFFICINALIS

Native of the Mediterranean region and cultivated in other areas, it grows to about 6 ft (2 m) high, with woody stems and needle-like leaves. The pale lilac or blue flowers have a distinctive scent.

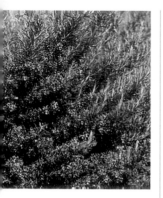

How it Works in the Body

- The combined constituents of rosemary, including the apigenin, rosmarinic, and ursolic acids have an anti-inflammatory action:
- The diosmetin is known to help in strengthening the capillaries, which is valuable in the cardiovascular system.
- Used to improve circulation and raise low blood pressure.
- Believed to improve memory and concentration.
- Also used in Reynaud's Syndrome, a condition of poor circulation in the hands and feet.
- Sometimes used to improve states of lethargy and debility.

Applications

Infusion Take 8 fl oz (200 ml) daily, internally. Externally, use as a rinse for the hair to improve circulation to the scalp and encourage hair growth. Add to a bath.

Tincture Take 40 drops (2 ml) twice a day.

Essential oil Add to bathwater or use in a diffuser to aid concentration.

Parts used

Leaves, essential oil.

Active constituents

Volatile oil, flavonoids, including apigenin and diosmetin, rosmarinic acid and other phenolic acids, diterpenes, triterpenes, including ursolic acid.

Indications

- Memory loss and poor concentration.
- Cold hands and feet from poor circulation.
- Low blood pressure.
- States of debility.
- Baldness or receding hair line.

Contraindications

- This herb should not be used if you suffer from high blood pressure.

Yellow Dock

Polygonaceae RUMEX CRISPUS

Also called curled dock due to the shape of the leaves which have furled edges. It is largely found in wastelands and at the roadside. Its origins are in Europe and Africa, but it is cultivated everywhere.

How it Works in the Body

- The anthraquinones are responsible for the laxative effect for which this herb is mainly used:
- They stimulate the colon to expel waste and toxins. In small amounts anything that has a laxative effect may be cleansing for the body. At the right dosage the plant gives a gentle action well-suited to relieveing moderate constipation.* It also acts to aid the digestive processes.
- Combined with other herbs, yellow dock can assist the liver in the cleansing of toxins from the skin, and is used in complaints such as eczema, psoriasis, and acne.
- In the musculoskeletal system, where there is often a buildup of toxins resulting from constipation, the herb is again cleansing.

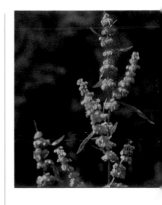

Applications

Decoction Use the root. Take 4 fl oz (100 ml) daily for short periods for constipation. For skin problems, combine with marigold and cleavers and use 4 fl oz (100 ml) daily of the three herbs combined.

Tincture Take 50 drops (2½ ml) three times a day.

Parts used

Root.

Active constituents

Anthraquinone glycosides, tannins, rumicin, and oxalates.

Indications

- Constipation and poor digestion.
- Skin complaints such as eczema, psoriasis, and acne.
- Arthritic complaints.
- Fungal infections.

Contraindications

- **Do not** take during pregnancy or while breastfeeding.

**Large amounts of yellow dock would have a purgative effect, causing excessive peristalsis, resulting in griping pains.*

Sage

Labiatae SALVIA OFFICINALIS

Also called garden, or red sage, it comes from the Mediterranean regions and has with paired, wrinkled, reddish purple leaves. The leaves, when crushed, have a distinctive odor.

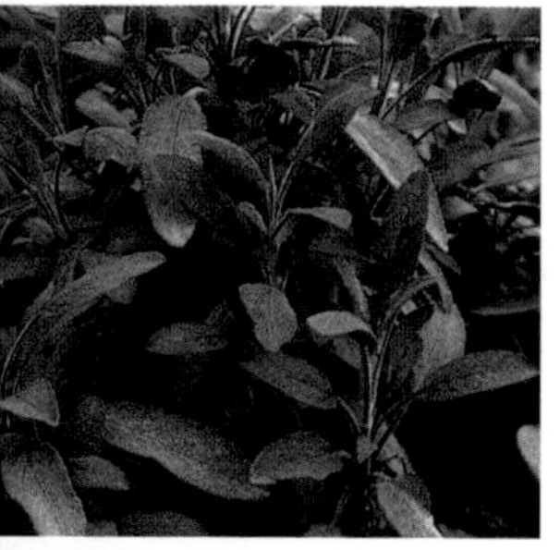

How it Works in the Body

- The thujone is mainly responsible for sage's antiseptic properties, which makes it invaluable for use both as a gargle and a mouthwash.
- It also acts as a circulatory and mild digestive stimulant.
- In the reproductive system, sage can be used to bring on a delayed period, and in menopause can be taken to relieve sweats and balance hormonal changes.
- Rosmarinic acid acting as an anti-inflammatory and anti-spasmodic properties.

Applications

Infusion 8 fl oz (200 ml) a day, or use as a gargle or mouthwash, 4 fl oz (100 ml), two to three times a day. (See Herbal Methods chapter, gargles and mouthwashes p.32).

Tincture Take 40 drops (2 ml), twice a day.

Parts used

Leaves.

Active constituents

Volatile oil with thujone, cineole, borneol and camphor, diterpene bitters, flavonoids, phenolic acids (e.g. rosmarinic), and salviatannin.

Indications

- Sore or bleeding gums.
- Mouth ulcers, sore throats, tonsillitis, and similar problems.
- Poor circulation and digestion.
- Delayed period.
- Menopause.

Contraindications

- **Do not** take during pregnancy.

Elderflower

Caprifoliaceae SAMBUCUS NIGRA

The elder grows in woods and on wasteground in Europe. When flowering it is a mass of creamy-white, flat-topped blossoms, which are followed by bunches of black berries.

How it Works in the Body

- The herb has an anti-inflammatory action, attributed to the presence of the ursolic acid. It mostly benefits the respiratory system.
- Useful for allergies, hayfever and allergic rhinitis.
- It has a diaphoretic effect, which encourages the loss of toxins through sweating, so it is particularly useful in colds and flu, where it will lower a fever and reduce excess catarrh.
- Relieves earache where this is due to the buildup of mucus.
- It has a mild diuretic effect on the urinary system, encouraging the elimination of waste, helpful in arthritic conditions.

Parts used

Flowers, berries, leaves, bark.

Active constituents

Triterpenes (including ursolic acid), fixed oils, flavonoids, phenolic acids.

Applications

Infusion Drink 8 fl oz (200 ml), three times a day as a mouthwash. Use in the bath to soothe dry skin, and to clear blocked sinuses.
Tincture Take 1 tsp (5 ml), three times a day.
Decoction Take 8 fl oz (200 ml) twice a day.
Ointment Use for chilblains, wounds, and dry skin.

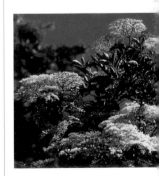

Indications

- Coughs and colds.
- Sore throats.
- Dry skin.
- Chilblains and wounds.
- Arthritic conditions.

Contraindications

- None.

Skullcap

Labiatae SCUTELLARIA LATERIFLORA

Native to North America, skullcap is also found in Europe, but the variety has different medicinal qualities. The plant has thin stems covered in hairs and blue flowers. The seed capsules give the herb its name, being shaped like a cap.

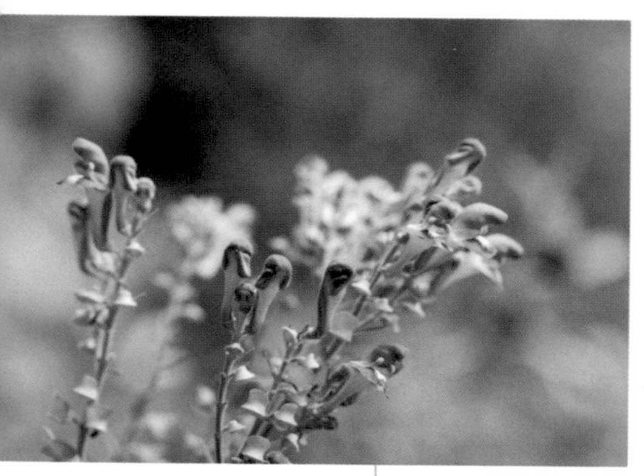

How it Works in the Body

- Skullcap works mainly on the nervous system, acting as a sedative, both mentally and physically, to calm and sustain an overexcited system.
- Can be effective to relieve stress and tension.
- Some species of skullcap contain constituents which have anti-inflammatory and anti-allergenic properties.
- A species found in China has a beneficial effect in liver disorders such as hepatitis.
- Skullcap's sedative effect also helps to alleviate period or ovarian pain.

Parts used

Whole herb.

Active constituents

Flavonoid glycoside, scutellarin, iridoids, volatile oils and waxes, tannins.

Applications

Infusion 8 fl oz (200 ml) three times a day.

Tincture 40 drops (2 ml) three times a day.

Indications

- Stress and anxiety.
- Insomnia (use alongside passionflower).
- Inflammation and allergic reactions.
- Ovarian and period pain.
- Liver disorder.

Contraindications

- None.

Saw Palmetto

Palmaceae SERENOA SERRULATA/SABAL SERRULATA

This plant originates from North America and is a palm that grows to about 9 ft (3 m), with large, fanned-out leaves. The flowers are pale and the fruit a deep reddish-brown.

How it Works in the Body

- Saw palmetto is a tonic that builds and restores body tissue.
- Sterols have an anabolic action, which helps to build and maintain weight, so it is useful for those who are convalescing or have lost weight through illness or debility.
- In the reproductive system it has useful applications for both men and women. In men it can be given to enhance sex drive and to treat impotence and infertility.
- In women it is thought to have an estrogenic action and can be used to assist the reproductive system.
- As a urinary tract tonic it is used where there is weakness in the bladder, and also as a diuretic to improve urinary flow.
- Saw palmetto has been shown to be effective in treating enlargement of the prostate.

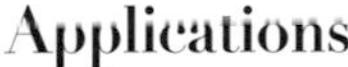

Applications

Infusion 4 fl oz (100 ml) twice daily.

Tincture 40 drops (2 ml) three times a day.

Parts used

Berries.

Active constituents

Essential oil, fixed oil, sterols, polysaccharides.

Indications

- Weight loss due to illness.
- Low sex drive and impotence in men.
- Low estrogenic levels in women.
- Urinary tract ailments.
- Enlarged prostate.

Contraindications

- None.

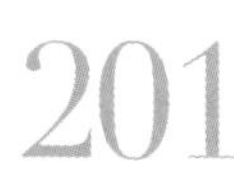

Chickweed

Caryophyllaceae STELLARIA MEDIA

Chickweed is a common garden weed originating in Europe and it now grows worldwide. The plant grows close to the ground, with dark-green, oval leaves and has tiny, white, star-like flowers.

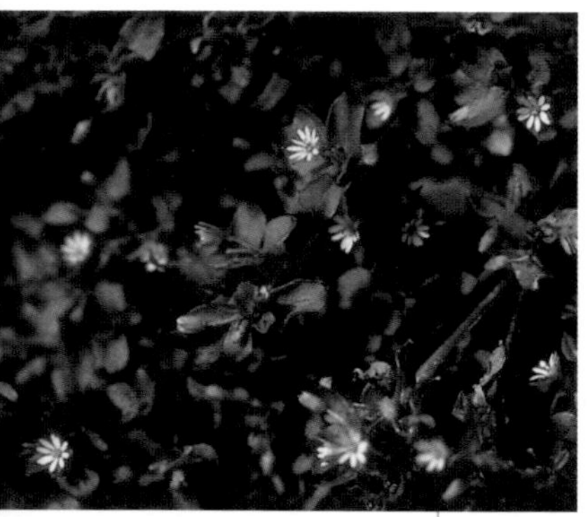

How it Works in the Body

- The saponins in chickweed are responsible for the relief of itching.
- Saponins have a cooling quality, and are especially soothing when applied to hot and itchy skin.
- Useful on wounds to reduce scarring.
- Beneficial for arthritic conditions.
- Topically the whole plant has a soothing, healing quality.
- Can also be used to aid the digestive system when taken in small amounts, soothing and healing the digestive tract.

Applications

Infusion Take 8 fl oz (200 ml) twice a day, or use in the bath.

Cream or ointment Use twice a day, or as a poultice if required.

Tincture Use internally, 20 drops (1 ml) three times a day.

Parts used

The leaves and flowers together.

Active constituents

Saponin glycosides, coumarins, flavonoids, carboxylic acids, triterpenoids, and vitamin C.

Indications

- Eczema, psoriasis, and irritative skin complaints.
- Wounds with possible scarring.
- Boils and abscesses.
- Arthritic complaints, pain and stiffness.
- Sore throats and coughs.
- Irritated, upset digestive system.
- Diarrhea.

Contraindications

- This herb may have a laxative effect in large doses.
- **Avoid** during pregnancy.

Comfrey

Boraginaceae SYMPHYTUM OFFICINALE

The main feature of this plant is the leaves. The plant itself grows to about 3 ft (1 m) high and the leaves are large, oval, and bristly. The flowers are drooping and bell-like, either white or purple.

How it Works in the Body

- Allantoin, the principal ingredient in comfrey, works to promote the healing of tissues within the body. It is complemented by the rosmarinic acid, an anti-inflammatory agent.
- Mucilage is demulcent and works to soothe irritative conditions, both internally and externally.
- Tannins act as an astringent.
- Pyrrolizidine alkaloids are thought to be damaging to the liver. These are mainly concentrated in the root of the plant, and therefore should not be taken internally.

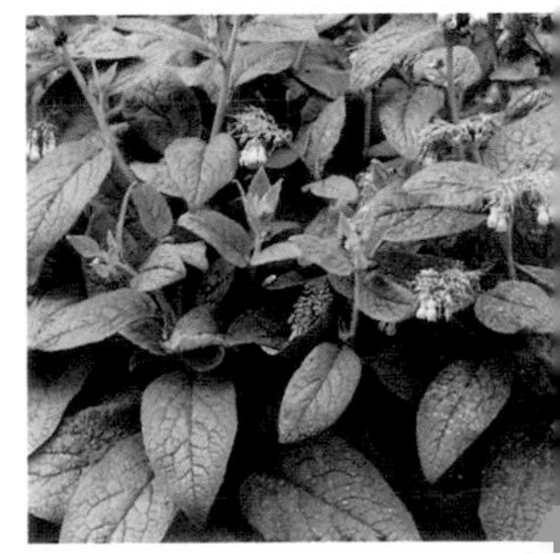

Applications

Tincture Only use the leaf.
Poultice or compress Made from the leaf.
Infused oil Made from the leaf; can be used as a massage oil.
Ointment May be used instead of the oil.

Indications

- Stomach ulcers and irritable bowel syndrome.
- Bronchitic conditions.
- Injury, sprains, breaks, and bruises.
- Arthritic joints.
- Scar tissue

Contraindications

- Never take the leaf without the supervision of a qualified herbal or medical practitioner. Never take the root internally.
- Never apply any comfrey preparations to an open wound, cut, or graze.

Parts used

Leaf, internally. Root, externally.

Active constituents

Allantoin, pyrrolizidine alkaloids, phenolic acids including rosmarinic, mucilage, volatile oil, tannins, and saponins.

Feverfew

Compositae TANACETUM PARTHENIUM

Feverfew grows to about 2 ft (60 cm) and is daisy-like in appearance, with yellow, central florets surrounded by an outer ring of white. The leaves are yellowish green and fern-like.

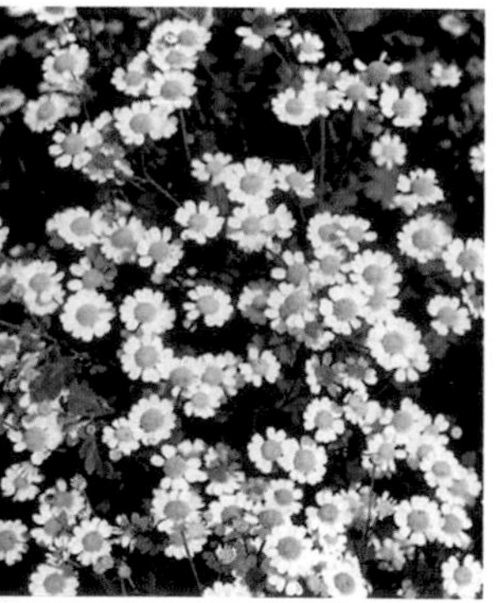

How it Works in the Body

- Feverfew's action against fevers is thought to be due to the sesquiterpene lactones, which inhibit the release of arachidonic acid in the body.
- In the reproductive system, feverfew has an age-old function of promoting menstrual flow.
- Mainly used to prevent and alleviate headaches, especially migraine. The sesquiterpene lactones, among the other constituents, are thought to inhibit the secretion of serotonin, which is implicated in the onset of migraine.
- In the musculoskeletal system, its inhibitory effects are thought to help control pain in conditions such as arthritis.

Applications

The fresh leaf Take two leaves daily wrapped in a piece of bread.

Tincture 10 drops (½ ml) once a day.

Tablets Available commercially. Use stated dosage.

Part used

Leaves.

Active constituents

Volatile oil containing spiroketal enol ethers; sesquiterpene lactones including parthenolide; acetylene derivatives, mainly in the root.

Indications

- Fevers.
- Delayed or painful periods.
- Headaches, especially migraine.
- Arthritic conditions.

Contraindications

- **Do not** take during pregnancy.
- **Never** take this herb if you take Warfarin or other blood-thinning medication.
- The fresh leaf may cause ulcers if eaten on its own without bread.

Pao d'Arco

Bignoniaceae TABEBUIA SPECIES

There are many different species of Pao d'Arco (its Portuguese name) or lapacho (its Spanish name). The tree grows to about 100 ft (30 m), and has pinkish-purple flowers.

How it Works in the Body

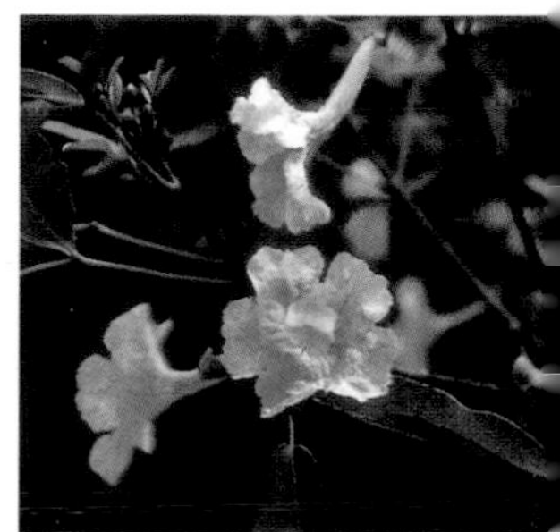

- Lapachol has an anti-bacterial action which makes Pao d'Arco a valuable natural antibiotic.
- Anti-fungal properties of the herb are effective against ringworm, vaginal thrush, and gastrointestinal candidiasis.
- Carnosol is a strong antioxidant which mops up free radicals in the body.
- A form of lapachone has an antiviral action and has been used against cold sores.
- Alkaloids can benefit diabetes sufferers and its detoxifying element is used in skin complaints.
- Its anti-inflammatory action is helpful for conditions such as cystitis, prostatitis, and intestinal inflammation.

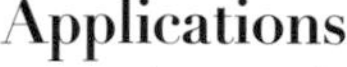

Applications

Decoction Drink 8 fl oz (200 ml) three times a day.

Tincture Take 60 drops (3 ml) three times a day. Soak a tampon in a strong infusion of the herb and insert as usual.

Tablets Available commercially. Use stated dosage.

Indications

- Bacterial and viral infection in ear, nose, and throat.
- Vaginal thrush and candidiasis in gastrointestinal tract.
- Cystitis, prostatitis, and stomach inflammation.
- Flu and colds.

Contraindications

- None.

Part used

Inner bark.

Active constituents

The main active ingredient in this plant is the quinones, of which there are eighteen, the main ones being naphthoquinones, of which lapachol and a form of lapachone are some of the most important. Other consituents are the bioflavonoid quercetin, lapachenole, carnosol, indoles, coenzyme Q, alkaloids, and steroidal saponins.

Dandelion

Compositae TARAXACUM OFFICINALE *(pu gong ying)*

The shiny leaves are noted for their jagged, tooth-like shape. The flowers are bright yellow. This well-known weed grows on wasteland and cultivated areas alike. Originating in Europe and Asia, it now grows in many countries.

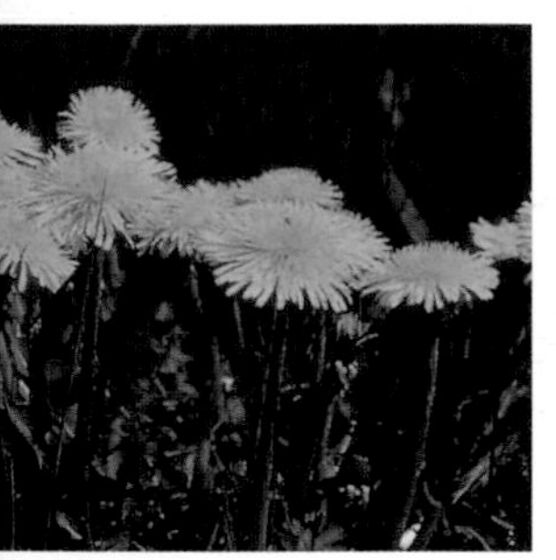

How it Works in the Body

- Dandelion leaves contain a high amount of potassium, which balances their function as a powerful diuretic.
- The root functions differently, being used to treat the liver to improve its function, and as a mild laxative.
- Both leaf and root act as a tonic to the gallbladder. Its detoxifying properties remove the effects of pollution on the body.
- In women who are breastfeeding, it is used to promote lactation.
- Also used to boost appetite.

Parts used

Leaves and root.

Active constituents

Sesquiterpene lactones, triterpenes, phenolic acids, polysaccharides, carotenoids, and vitamins A and C, potassium.

Applications

Fresh Use in salads or soups; add to tonic wines.
Infusion Use the leaf; 8 fl oz (200 ml) three times daily.
Tincture Take 40 drops (2 ml) three times daily.
Decoction Use the root in a decoction. Take 8 fl oz (200 ml) twice a day.

Indications

- Water retention and high blood pressure.
- Arthritic, kidney and liver conditions.
- Eczema, psoriasis, and acne.
- Gallstones.
- Excessive alcohol consumption.

Contraindications

- None.

Thyme

Labiatae THYMUS VULGARIS

There are a huge number of species of thyme. Common or garden thyme is a native of the Mediterranean and cultivated in many parts of the world. Wild thyme is native to Europe.

How it Works in the Body

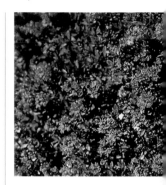

- Primarily used a remedy for the respiratory system. Tymol has expectorant and antiseptic qualities, invaluable for chest infections and respiratory ailments.
- Can be used in the urinary tract as an antiseptic, and acts with other constituents as an anti-spasmodic.
- It has a sedative effect useful for asthma and hayfever.
- It also has an anti-larval action.
- The oil can be used as a counter-irritant, to draw blood to a cold joint in cases of rheumatic disorder.

Applications

Infusion Take 8 fl oz (200 ml) twice a day.

Tincture Take 40 drops (2 ml) three times daily.

Syrup Use with licorice, take 2 tsp (10 ml) three times daily.

Essential oil Combine in a base oil, or take on its own, two drops in 4 tbsp (50 ml) base oil as a rub. Add to water as an inhalation.

Indications

- Respiratory complaints, such as asthma, bronchitis, hayfever, sore throats, and coughs.
- Arthritic complaints, cold joints, tired and aching muscles.
- Urinary tract infections (in combination with other herbs).
- Worms.

Parts used

Whole herb, essential oil.

Active constituents

Volatile oil, especially thymol, with cineole, borneol and others, flavonoids, caffeic acid, tannins.

Contraindications

- **Do not** use during pregnancy.

Lime Blossom

Tiliaceae TILIA EUROPAEA

Lime blossom, or limeflower as it is also known, is the flower of the linden tree which grows to a height of 100 ft (30 m). It has heart-shaped leaves and yellowish-white flowers, which hang in clusters.

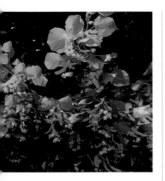

How it Works in the Body

- The relaxing qualities of lime blossom make it extremely useful in the nervous system, for conditions requiring an anti-spasmodic action.
- Helpful as a remedy for sleeplessness due to its sedative action.
- For headaches, especially caused by excess catarrh.
- Lime blossom is used to treat high blood pressure, and to lower cholesterol associated with arteriosclerosis.
- Useful for indigestion associated with nervous tension.
- Has a diaphoretic action, which helps the body to sweat out toxins.

Applications

Infusion Use 8 fl oz (200 ml) three times a day for indigestion, stress, headaches, and general tension. It can be added to bath water to calm and relax.

Tincture Take between ½–1 tsp (2–5 ml) at bedtime for sleeplessness. Take 40 drops (2 ml) three times a day for high blood pressure.

Parts used

Flowers.

Active constituents

Volatile oil, flavonoids, mucilage, phenolic acids, tannins.

Indications

- Indigestion and stress-related stomach complaints.
- Insomnia.
- Headaches, especially where there is excess catarrh.
- Symptoms of colds and flu.
- High blood pressure, to lower cholesterol levels.

Contraindications

Do not use this herb for low blood pressure.

Coltsfoot

Compositae TUSSILAGO FARFARA *(kuan dong hua)*

The plant has a flowering stem with star-like, yellow flowers and broad green leaves. It originated in Europe and Asia and now grows extensively in North America.

How it Works in the Body

- Flavonoids have an antispasmodic and anti-inflammatory effect, which eases spasm in the lungs during asthma and bronchitis attacks.
- Polysaccharides are anti-inflammatory, which helps to calm irritated lung tissue. They also act as an expectorant for excess phlegm and mucus.
- Constituents work to improve the immune system and promote a healthy respiratory system.
- Pyrrolizidine alkaloids are thought to be harmful to the liver, but to a large extent are destroyed when prepared as a decoction.

Part used
Leaves.

Active constituents
Flavonoids, mucilage (about 8 per cent, consisting mainly of polysaccharides), pyrrolizidine alkaloids, tannin.

Applications

Decoction The herb is prepared as a decoction for the treatment of coughs and other chest complaints.
Tincture Take 1 ml (20 drops) twice daily to improve the lungs. It is particularly good for coughs when used as a syrup. The Chinese dosage is 1/16–1/2 oz (1.5–9 g).

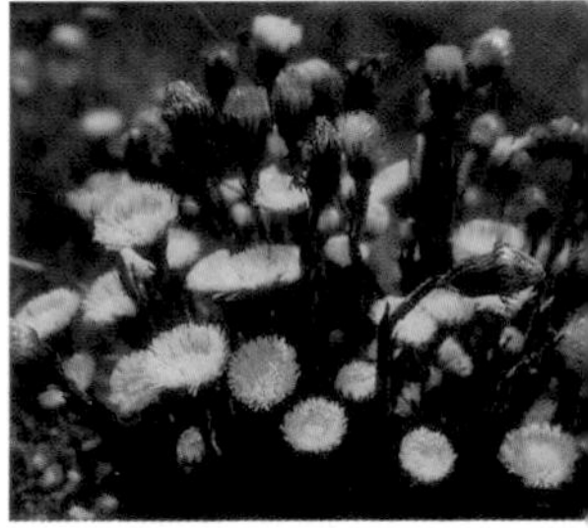

Indications

- Dry and irritating coughs.
- To generally improve the health of the lungs where there are lung complaints, such as asthma or bronchitis.

Contraindications

- Only use the leaves, not the flowers.
- **Do not** take while pregnant or during breastfeeding.
- **Do not** give to children under six years old.

Stinging Nettle

Urticaceae URTICA DIOICA

The nettle grows to 4 ft (1.2 m) and it has serrated green leaves, the flowers grow in clusters. The main feature of the nettle is its covering of fine hairs, which can sting.

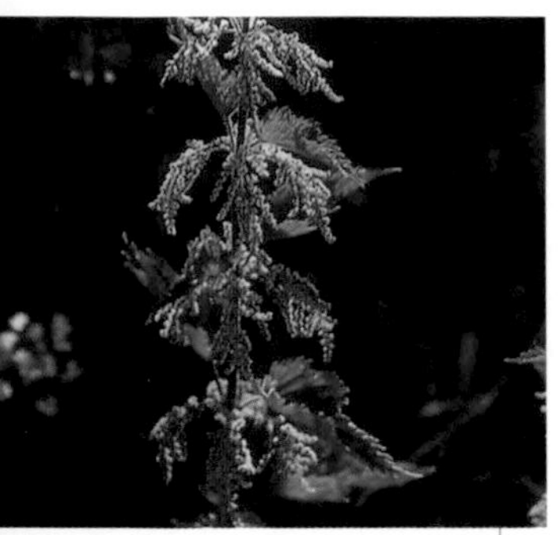

How it Works in the Body

- Nettle loses its stinging effect when subjected to heat, either in cooking or when made into an infusion.
- Used to treat skin complaints as an antiallergenic, and can be used to treat eczema and related allergies when taken internally.
- It is antihemorrhagic and can be used as an astringent to stop excessive bleeding from wounds, or in the reproductive system.
- Iron and vitamin C in the nettle are an excellent tonic for anemia and lack of iron.
- Root can be used to treat an enlarged prostate.

Applications

Infusion Take 8 fl oz (200 ml) twice daily.

Decoction of the roots 8 fl oz (200 ml) daily.

Tincture Take 60 drops (3 ml) three times a day.

Soup Use the young tops of the leaves, picked in spring. Take as a daily tonic.

Parts used

Herb and root.

Active constituents

Chlorophyll, indoles (e.g. histamine and serotonin), acetylcholine, vitamin C, iron, and dietary fiber.

Indications

- Skin conditions, such as eczema.
- Allergic conditions, hayfever, and asthma.
- Iron deficiency.
- Heavy bleeding.
- Enlargement of the prostate.

Contraindications

- A small number of people find that irritation occurs when ingesting nettle. If this happens, discontinue use and consult a doctor.

Valerian

Valerianaceae VALERIANA OFFICINALIS

The plant grows to about 3 ft (1 m) high. It flourishes in wet and marshy conditions and is often found near rivers. The leaves occur in pairs and the flowers are pale pink or white, with a distinctive smell.

How it Works in the Body

- Valerian's usefulness in the nervous system is mainly due to the valepotriates, which have a sedative effect on the mind.
- Used to treat insomnia, helping the sufferer to fall asleep more quickly and wake in the morning without feeling stupefied.
- Helpful for all types of stress-related anxiety as it does not impair the ability to concentrate, but has a calming effect.
- Can be used to treat numerous ailments, including digestive complaints where there is a contributing stress or tension factor.
- Acts as a muscle relaxant, and is used with other herbs in the cardiovascular system to treat high blood pressure.

Applications

Decoction Take 4 fl oz (100 ml) twice daily. For insomnia take 8 fl oz (200 ml) at night.

Tincture Taken 40 drops (2 ml) three times a day.

Tablets Available commercially. Use stated dosage.

Parts used
Root.

Active constituents
Volatile oil containing valerenic acid, iridoids known as valepotriates, alkaloids, flavonoids, sterols, and tannins.

Indications

- Insomnia, especially where there is overactivity of the mind.
- Stress and anxiety for short periods.
- Digestive complaints where stress is a factor, in combination with other herbs.
- High blood pressure

Contraindications

- A few people find this herb stimulating. If so, discontinue use.
- Large dose may cause stomach ache and mental sluggishness.

Crampbark

Caprifoliaceae VIBURNUM OPULUS/PRUNIFOLIUM

Crampbark is a shrub which grows to approximately 9 ft (3 m) and belongs to the same family as the elder tree. It is commonly found in woods and hedges.

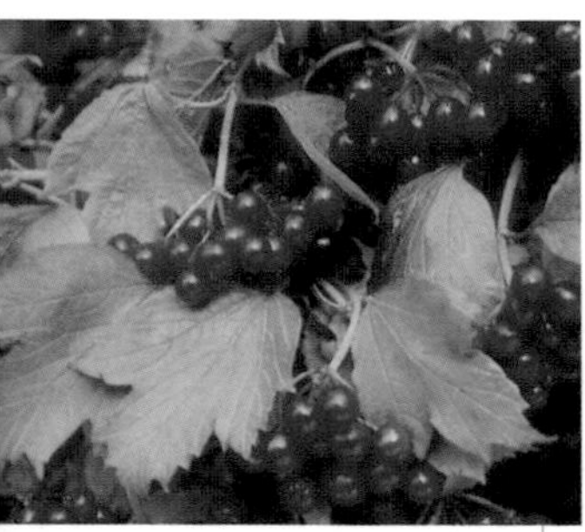

How it Works in the Body

- Crampbark acts as a muscle relaxant. The *opulus* variety is thought to act on the body as a whole, while the *prunifolium* variety acts particularly to relax the muscles of the uterus.
- Relieves the cramps that occur during a period.
- In the stomach it can relieve symptoms of irritable bowel syndrome.
- Can help to relax the airways in asthma and relieve arthritic pain.
- Helps to reduce high blood pressure.

Applications

Decoction Take when spasm is present. Take 4 fl oz (100 ml) up to six times daily.

Tincture Take when spasm is present. Take 50 drops (3 ml) up to six times a day. For external relief of muscle spasm, add 40 drops (2 ml) of the tincture to 1½ oz (30 g) cream, e.g. comfrey, and mix well. Apply up to three times a day.

Parts used

Bark from branches—only use small amounts at any one time as the removal of large amounts of bark may kill the tree.

Active constituents

Hydroquinones, coumarins, tannins.

Indications

- Uterine and ovarian (period) cramps.
- Arthritic cramps.
- Muscle tension, spasm and night cramps.
- High blood pressure.
- Asthma.

Contraindications

- **Do not** take this remedy during pregnancy.
- **Do not** take if you have low blood pressure.

Chaste Berry

Verbenaceae VITEX AGNUS-CASTUS

Chaste berry is a shrub that grows to about 20 ft (7 m). The leaves have five to seven leaflets, dark-green on top and gray beneath, with small, purple flowers and an aromatic fragrance.

How it Works in the Body

- Chaste berry has different, distinct actions for men or women. In men it acts to depress the male androgen hormones, responsible for the male sex drive and so is rarely given to men.
- In women it affects the pituitary gland, which sends chemical messages to regulate the hormone balance in the body, including the two main hormones, estrogen and progesterone.
- Invaluable in treating many disorders in the reproductive system that are due to an imbalance of these hormones, for example, PMS, irregular periods, and infertility. It can also be used to treat acne.

Parts used

Berries.

Active constituents

Iridoid glycosides (including aucibin and agnoside), volatile oil (cineol), fixed oils, alkaloids (viticine), and flavonoids (casticin).

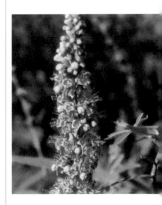

Applications

Tincture Take 20 drops (1 ml) in water first thing in the morning daily, increasing to 40 drops (2 ml) if needed.
Tablets Available commercially. Use stated dosage.

Indications

- Hormonal imbalance and related conditions.
- PMS (mood swings, bloating, breast tenderness).
- Irregular periods.
- Migraine associated with the menstrual cycle.
- Acne.

Contraindications

- None.

Maize (Cornsilk)

Gramineae ZEA MAYS *(yu mi xu)*

This plant now grows in warm climates throughout the world. The cornsilk refers to the fronds that surround the corn cob. Once the female flower has been fertilized these turn brown and yellow kernels grow beneath them.

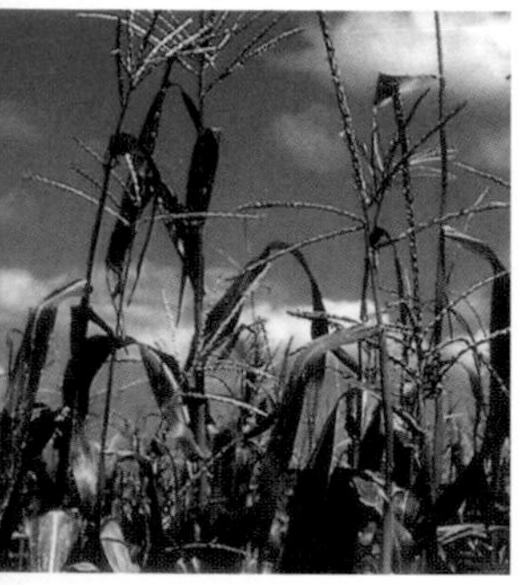

How it Works in the Body

- Maize works mainly in the urinary tract.
- Saponins largely act as an anti-inflammatory in the body.
- Allantoin acts as a healing agent, with the mucilage giving a demulcent or soothing effect to irritated tissues.
- Potassium balances out the diuretic effect of the herb, which is useful to treat water retention.
- Useful for a number of urinary tract conditions, such as cystitis and prostatitis.
- Vitamin K is a fat-soluble vitamin that is essential for blood clotting within the body.

Applications

Infusion, fresh or dried Take 8 fl oz (200 ml) three times a day.

Decoction Use as a poultice for wounds and sores.

Tincture Take 50 drops (3 ml) three times a day for conditions such as cystitis.

Parts used

Cornmeal (kernels) externally, cornsilk internally.

Active constituents

Saponins, allantoin, sterols, alkaloid (hordenine), mucilage, vitamins C and K, and potassium.

Indications

- Water retention.
- High blood pressure.
- Frequent urination, e.g. cystitis.
- Difficulty in passing water, e.g. prostatitis.
- Kidney problems, e.g. kidney stones.

Contraindications

- **Do not** take if you suffer from low blood pressure.

Ginger

Zingiberaceae ZINGIBER OFFICINALE *(sheng jiang)*

The aerial part of the plant consists of a green stalk with narrow leaves and a spike of yellow or white flowers. The root or rhizome has the long, tuberous joints familiar in cooking.

How it Works in the Body

- Phenolic compounds are the agents responsible for relaxing the muscles of the stomach. Fresh or dried, the root has been shown to minimize vomiting and ease travel or motion sickness.
- The phenolic ingredients act within the stomach as a sedative and painkiller, which helps to reduce overactivity of the gut.
- Oil acts as an antiseptic and an anti-inflammatory in the stomach.
- The gingerols alone are thought to be responsible for ginger's action as a liver protective.
- Ginger is thought to also reduce cholesterol levels, while at the same time increasing a sluggish circulation.

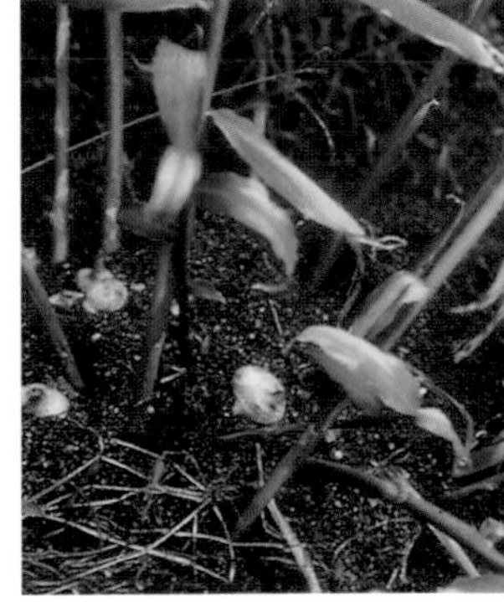

Applications

Infusion 8 fl oz (200 ml) three times a day.

Tincture Take 20 drops (1 ml) three times a day to improve the circulation, and for coughs, colds, and flu symptoms.

Indications

- Travel and motion sickness.
- Indigestion and nausea.
- Sickness in pregnancy.
- Sluggish/poor circulation.
- High cholesterol.
- Colds, flu, and coughs.
- Over-activity of the gut, wind, and bloating.

Parts used

Root or rhizome.

Active constituents

Volatile oil, phenolic compounds, including gingerols and shogaols.

Contraindications

- Do not use for lung infections with fevers, or with irritative digestive complaints, such as ulcers and acid indigestion.

Additional Herbs

A brief description of herbs used or mentioned in the book but not listed in the Herbal Directory.

Agrimony *Agrimonia eupatoria* Astringent and tonic properties, making it a valuable remedy for the treatment of childhood diarrhea and urinary incontinence.

Arnica *Arnica montana* One of the best herbs for healing bruising and sprains. Do not use if skin is broken.

Bladderwrack *Fucus vesiculosus* Very useful for regulating the thyroid gland. Helps an underactive thyroid and goiter.

Boneset *Eupatorium perfoliatum* One of the best remedies for the relief of symptoms associated with flu—relieves fevers, catarrh, aches, and pains.

Borage *Borago officinalis* Benefits the adrenal glands, helping to restore function after the use of steroids. Also helps boost the immune system.

Bugleweed *Lycopus europaens* Specific use for overactive thyroid, helping with symptoms of palpitations, shaking, and breathing difficulties.

Catnip *Nepeta cataria* Traditionally used for the treatment of colds and flu, but also relaxing and calming properties. Especially suitable for children with fevers.

Cayenne *Capsicum minimum* Stimulant and tonic, helping circulatory and digestive disorders. Use in small amounts—approximately one quarter of recommended general dosage.

Celery seed *Apium graveolens* Antiseptic useful in treatment of urinary problems, and also with dandelion leaf in rheumatic conditions.

Cinnamon *Cinnamomum zeylanicum* Helps to relieve nausea and vomiting, and mild cases of diarrhea.

Cloves *Eugenia caryophyllus* Stimulant to the digestive system. Powerful local antiseptic and mild anesthetic, can also be used for toothache. **Caution:** Do not swallow the clove pieces.

Damiana *Turnera aphrodisiaca* Helps strengthen the nervous system, and useful as antidepressant. Strengthens the male reproductive system, thus enhancing libido.

Elecampane *Inula helenium* Helpful for treating irritating bronchial coughs, especially in children. Helps with bronchitis and emphysema and also helps clear copious catarrh.

False unicorn root *Chamaelirium luteum* One of the best tonics for the female reproductive system. Take as a decoction, 4 fl oz (100 ml), twice daily, or as a tincture, 15 drops, twice daily. **Caution:** Do not exceed the dose as large amounts may cause nausea or vomiting. **Do not** take in pregnancy.

Fennel *Foeniculum vulgare* Excellent remedy for colic and flatulence. Helps increase milk flow in breastfeeding.

Forskolin *Coleus forskohlii* Used to aid digestion, help reduce blood pressure, and improve circulation.

Golden rod *Solidago virgaurea* Helpful for treating coughs, colds, and sinusitus. Useful for clearing catarrh in acute and chronic cases.

Horsetail *Equisetum arvense* Diuretic and astringent helpful in the treatment of urinary disorders, including bedwetting and incontinence.

Hyssop *Hyssopus officinalis*
Helps relieve coughs and colds. Also used as a relaxant for anxiety and hysteria.

Juniper berries
Juniperus communis
Excellent remedy for cystitis. Also used externally to ease painful muscles and joints. Do not take in pregnancy or with kidney disease.

Milk thistle *Silybum marianum*
Aid to the liver, helping to promote the flow of bile. Excellent remedy to promote milk flow when breastfeeding.

Myrrh *Commiphora molmol*
Strong anti-microbial action used for the treatment of infections, particularly as mouthwash.

Pilewort *Ranunculus ficaria*
Used specifically to treat hemorrhoids or piles. Use internally as a tea, or externally as an ointment.

Pokeroot *Phytolacca americana*
Valuable remedy to clear catarrh and cleanse the lymph system. **Caution:** In large doses pokeroot acts as a purgative.

Prickly ash bark and berries
Zanthoxylum americanum
Stimulating tonic for the circulatory system. Helpful for complaints such as poor circulation, varicose veins, and cramps.

Raspberry leaves *Rubus ideaus*
Toning for the womb. Caution: Use only during the last three months of pregnancy.

Red clover *Trifolium pratense*
Useful remedy for childhood eczema and hyperactivity, helps to cleanse the system.

Slippery elm *Ulmus fulva*
Soothing herb for digestive complaints. Also used externally as a poultice to treat boils and abscesses. Take as decoction, using one-part powder to eight-parts water, or as tablets.

Stone root
Collinsonia canadensis
Mainly used in the treatment of stones or gravel in the urinary system and the gallbladder.

Tea tree *Melaleuca alternifolia*
Used for its antiseptic and anti-fungal properties. **Caution:** Can irritate the skin so use in a carrier/base oil for athlete's foot and insect bites.

Thuja *Thuja occidentalis*
Used externally to treat warts and fungal infections. **Caution:** Use internally only under professional supervision.

Vervain *Verbena officinalis*
Nervine tonic that will strengthen the nervous system while relaxing and easing tension. Useful for depression following influenza.

Wild oats *Avena sativa*
Bridge between food and medicine. Useful as general tonic for the nervous system, especially in cases of debility or exhaustion. Also used as an anti-depressant. Take as gruel, porridge, or tincture.

Wild yam *Dioscorea villosa* Valuable herb that has antispasmodic, anti-inflammatory, and antirheumatic properties, as well as many properties found in the contraceptive pill. Used for colic, painful periods, and arthritis.

Yellow dock *Rumex crispus*
Useful for skin complaints and in treating constipation. Promotes the flow of bile, and encourages the action of the gallbladder.

Kitchen Remedies

Basic ingredients found in nearly every kitchen can be used as herbal remedies. Listed below are some common ailments and kitchen remedies that can be used to treat them gently and effectively.

Colds and Flu To make a warming drink, combine 1 tsp (5 ml) lemon juice with one crushed clove of garlic, a tablespoon of honey, and a pinch of either powdered cinnamon or ginger, and pour on a cupful of hot water. The lemon juice is antiseptic and contains vitamin C to fight off a cold; the garlic is antibiotic, helps reduce catarrh, and is good for all kinds of infections; while the cinnamon or ginger are warming.

Toothache To ease an aching tooth until you can see a dentist, hold a clove in your mouth over the tooth and slowly nibble away at it. Do not use more than two cloves at any one time, and do not swallow the pieces. If you have clove oil, use one or two drops on a small piece of cotton and hold over the tooth to obtain relief. Repeat twice if needed. Cloves are both antiseptic and pain-killing.

Itching skin/eczema Ordinary porridge oats can be used to alleviate itching skin and heal eczema. Prepare a decoction of the oats, strain, and add the liquid to a lukewarm bath (see Herbal Methods section, pp.20–47). Externally, oats are soothing and healing to the skin as well as cleansing. Taken as porridge or as a juice, oats are nutritious and strengthen the nervous system, acting as an antidepressant, and also helping to reduce cholesterol.

Coughs and Sore Throats Take half an onion, sliced, and alternate the layers with sugar on a plate. Place a bowl over this and leave overnight before pouring off the juice, which makes an excellent cough syrup. Onions are both antiseptic and healing.

Diarrhea A simple but effective emergency treatment is to drink a cup of ordinary tea without milk or sugar. The tannins will coat the lining of the stomach and astringe it, relieving the symptoms. For children, dilute fresh lemon juice with water and add a little honey. If this condition persists you must seek additional help as you run the risk of dehydrating, which is potentially very serious.

Stings and bites To alleviate the pain use cold cider vinegar as a wash. To prevent insect bites, especially before going away on vacation, eat plenty of garlic, as it will dissuade insects from bothering you.

A Family Remedy Chest

A home herbal medicine chest can be prepared in addition to a conventional first-aid kit, but should not replace it. (A conventional kit will contain such necessities as bandages, scissors, and a thermometer.) The essentials can be supplemented by a range of herbal remedies that will enhance your family's well-being.

Tablets

Slippery elm A useful remedy that will ease diarrhea and gastric upsets. Also available as a powder.

Echinacea Invaluable for infections; antiviral and antibacterial.

Capsules

Garlic oil Use to combat infections. Take before and during a vacation to deter insect bites. For ear infections, open capsule, place two drops on a small piece of cotton, and place in the ear.

Creams

Arnica Use for bruises and sprains. Do not apply to broken skin. Discontinue use as soon as discoloration disappears.

Comfrey Use on skin area over sprains, strains, and fractures. Do not apply to broken skin.

Ointments

Calendula

Use for cuts and grazes. Ideal for children and may be used for diaper rash to protect the baby's skin.

Essential oils

Lavender Acts as pain-killer. Apply to mild burns after cooling for 10 minutes. Use neat on insect bites and stings. See Herbal Directory, p.189, for its many other uses.

Thyme

Use as inhalation (see p.35) to ease breathing, catarrh, or sinusitis. Add five drops to a bath to relieve tired and aching muscles.

Gel

Aloe Vera

Use gel or keep the fresh plant on hand and break a leaf off when needed. Heals cuts and scrapes. Also good as a treatment for sunburn and itchy skin.

Herbs

Which herbs you keep on hand will be entirely a matter of personal choice. Some suggestions might be, camomile to calm digestive upsets and aid sleep; elderflower for colds or flu, hayfever, etc.; lime blossom for poor sleep and shock; meadowsweet for an acid stomach, arthritic pains, and headaches; and nettle for allergies and heavy bleeding.

Glossary

A brief description of some of the terms used in this book.

Alterative
Acts as a blood cleanser.

Anodyne
Pain-killer.

Anti-allergenic
Helps reduce allergic reactions.

Anti-bacterial
Works against bacteria which cause infection.

Anticarcinogenic
Works against cancer.

Anti-catarrhal
Reduces excess catarrh.

Anticholesterol
Reduces cholesterol levels.

Antidepressant
Active against depression.

Antiemetic
Helps prevent vomiting.

Antifungal
Works against fungal infections.

Anti-hemorrhagic
Helps prevent bleeding.

Anti-inflammatory
Reduces inflammation.

Antioxidant
Helps prevent breakdown of tissues.

Antispasmodic
Reduces muscle spasm.

Antithrombotic
Reduces blood clotting levels.

Antiviral
Works against viruses that cause infection.

Antiseptic
Helps prevent infection.

Astringent
Coats the surface of the skin, reducing fluids and bleeding.

Carminative
Helps relieve indigestion.

Counter-irritant
Causes local irritation by drawing blood, thus acting as pain-reliever.

Decongestant
Eases congestion caused by excess mucus.

Demulcent
Coats surface, soothing and aiding healing.

Diaphoretic
Encourages removal of toxins through sweating.

Diuretic
Helps relieve water retention by encouraging urination.

Edema
Swelling of the tissues due to excess water retention.

Emmenagogue
Encourages menstruation by stimulating uterine muscles.

Emollient
Soothing to the skin.

Expectorant
Promotes cough reflex, aiding the expulsion of phlegm.

Exudate
Discharge from sore or wound.

Hemostatic
Reduces bleeding.

Hyperthyroid
Overactivity of the thyroid gland.

Hypoglycemic
Reduces blood sugar levels.

Laxative
Promotes mild bowel evacuation.

Mucilage
Gelatinous, demulcent, and soothing.

Neuralgia
Nerve pain or irritation.

Purgative
Promotes strong evacuation of the bowels.

Refrigerant
Cooling and pain-relieving.

Relaxant
Relaxes muscles.

Sedative
Reduces activity of the nervous system.

Soporific
Causes drowsiness or sleep.

Tonic
Re-balances and nourishes the system.

Topically
External use.

Vulnary
Wound-healer.

Index

Page numbers in **bold** refer to illustrations